The Healthy,
Happy Gut Cookbook

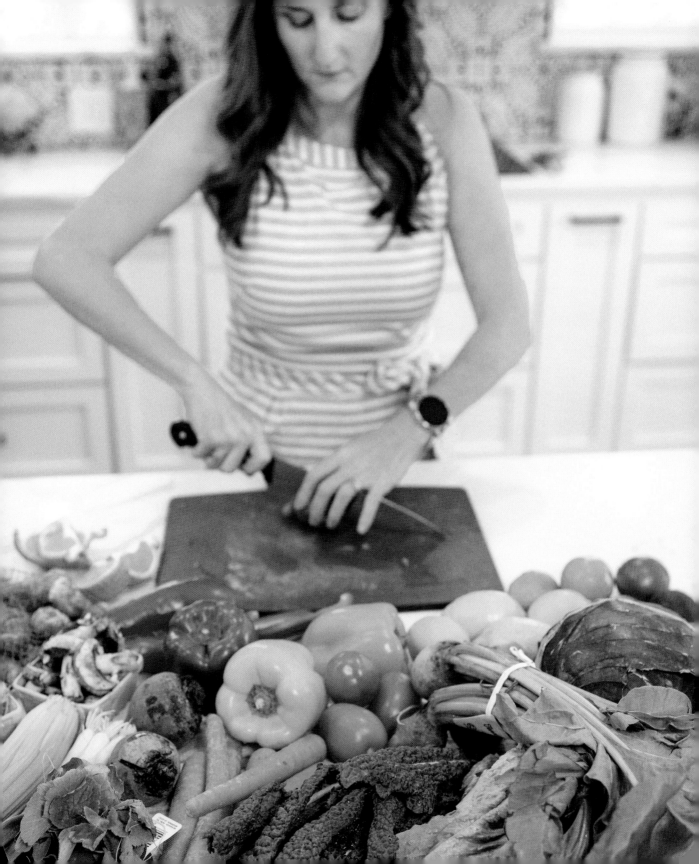

The Healthy, Happy Gut Cookbook

Simple, Non-Restrictive Recipes to Treat IBS,
Bloating, Constipation and Other Digestive
Issues the Natural Way

Dr. Heather Finley

Registered dietitian, gut health expert and
creator of the gutTogether™ method

PAGE STREET
PUBLISHING CO.

PAGE STREET
PUBLISHING CO.

Dedication

To my parents, for allowing me every opportunity to chase my dreams,

to my husband, for being the ultimate hype man,

and to Charlotte and Weldon—anything is possible!

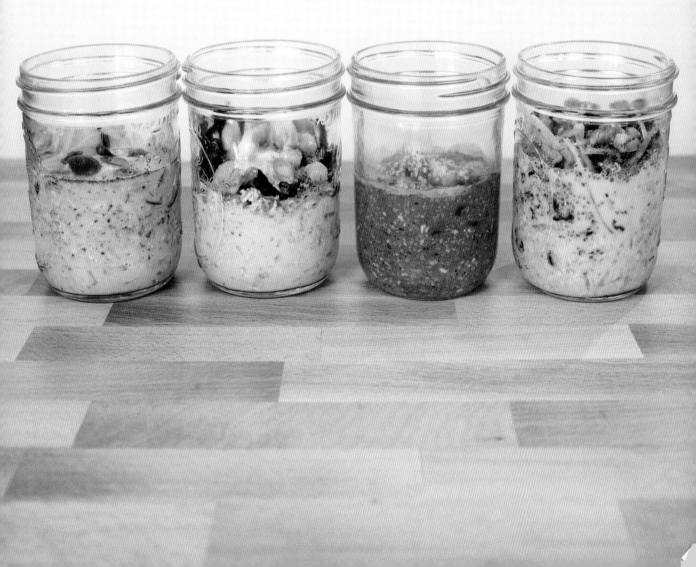

Table *of* Contents

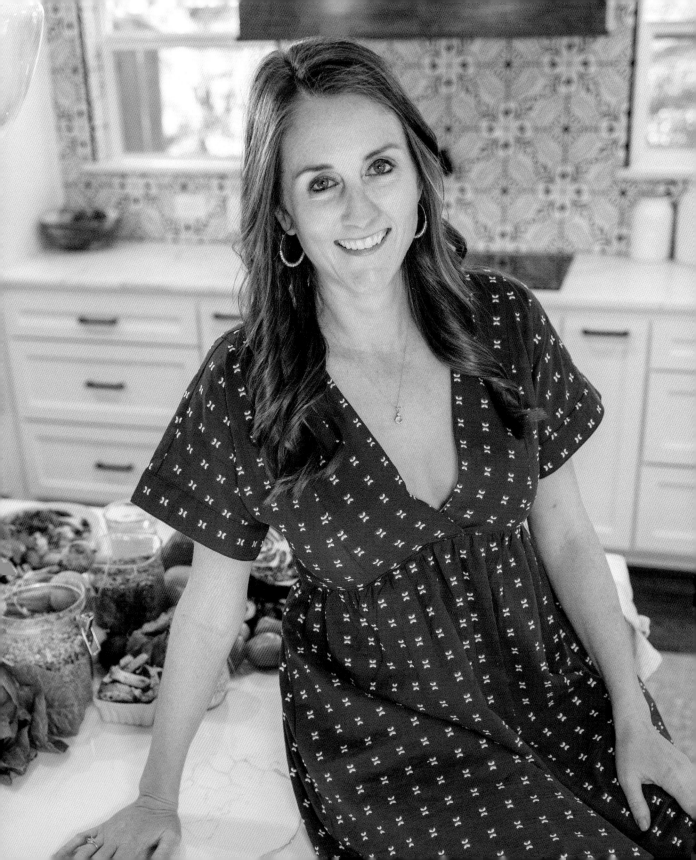

Introduction

My story, finding peace with food after 20 years of constipation

Your gut: the host of more than 100 trillion different bacteria, the location of digestion and absorption and the system that we continue to learn more about every day. I am excited you picked up this book! Maybe you did because you have been diagnosed with IBS (irritable bowel syndrome) or SIBO (small intestinal bacterial overgrowth). Maybe you don't have a diagnosis but you struggle with symptoms such as constipation, bloating, diarrhea, gas or food anxiety because of your digestive issues. Or maybe you feel like you have "tried everything" to resolve your gut symptoms and at this point you are starting to feel as though you will have to live with these symptoms indefinitely. I've been there, too.

The topic of gut health is quite trendy and somewhat of a buzzword these days. Every day we are learning more about how so many things (like mental health, skin health and even cardiovascular health) are connected back to the health of the gut.

Although your gut microbiota might not be a normal dinner conversation starter, I think by the end of this book you will have a newfound appreciation and admiration for it.

Your wonderful gut microbiota is made up of trillions of microbes that reside right inside of your intestines. Crazy, right? And what really blows my mind is that unlike our genes, we can impact the makeup of our gut by how we eat, how we move, how we sleep and even how we manage stress.

I struggled with chronic constipation for 20 years of my life. At times I thought to myself that it must just be normal to get bloated after eating anything, but later in life I learned that my struggle with constipation was anything but that. After years of hopping from one doctor to the next only to be told to "just eat more fiber" or "just take MiraLAX®," I decided to take matters into my own hands. I had a lightbulb moment while I was in my doctorate program that made me realize my constipation and bloat might not just be food related.

My years of elimination diets, restriction, overexercising and isolating myself from social events that involved food were in fact hurting my gut more than they were helping. At one point, I remember feeling as though there were only five foods that I could "safely" eat without bloating, gas or abdominal pain. I know that the thousands of clients I have worked with have felt this way, too, and maybe you do as well. I am here to help you dispel the food fear, improve your food variety and learn to fuel your gut with the diversity it craves (without a side of guilt!).

The years of digestive symptoms, food elimination and stress over my gut fueled my passion for helping as many people as possible get off the vicious-symptom cycle I was on for so many years. I hope that this book provides you with a new perspective and empowers you to take action toward improving your digestive symptoms.

Dr. Heather Finley

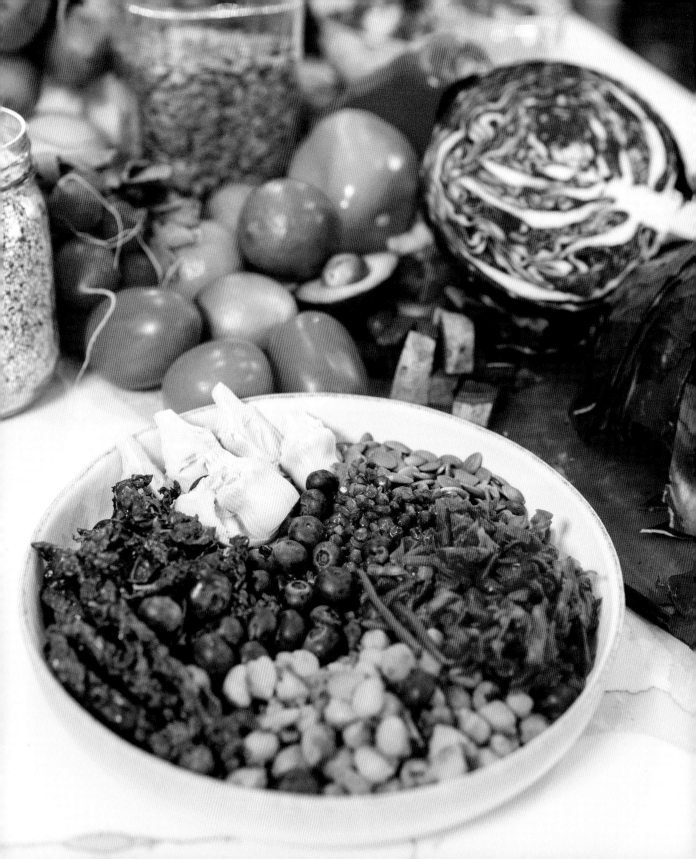

How to Use This Book

This book is meant to help you find sustainable relief from your digestive symptoms by slowly implementing strategies that become lifelong habits. This book is not a quick fix, fad or detox; to truly find long-term relief from your symptoms, the most important ingredients are consistency and time. This may be different than anything you have done before and may require you to really challenge your mindset about your symptoms, food and your body. We cover all of that in this book, and I hope that you finish reading feeling inspired, refreshed and encouraged that your digestive health journey does not have to involve extremes or fads.

To date, I have worked with more than 1,000 women in the gutTogether™ program, and there is one common theme I have observed. In today's wellness-obsessed world, the focus of digestive health is often backward. Instead of setting our intentions on sustainability and lifelong change, we are focused on the latest fad, detox or trend. This leaves people, just like you, feeling discouraged and as though they will never be "perfect" enough to find the relief they seek. I am here to change that narrative. Digestive health is not about restriction. It's about abundance, both in your life and on your plate. When you focus on the foundational habits that are emphasized in this book (and often overlooked in today's society), you can find relief with ease. You can rediscover the vibrancy you once had and live your life empowered in a way you have never known before.

This book will walk you step by step through the foundational habits necessary to promote digestive health and provide you with solutions that you might have not tried before. If you try to make all these changes at once, you will be overwhelmed. Instead, implement one change at a time and celebrate your successes along the way. Rather than focusing on all the changes that you have not been able to implement, celebrate everything that you have already implemented. This mindset shift can be powerful and will help sustain you as you take the next steps.

There is a useful guide in Appendix A on page 151 that will help you keep track of the sustainable changes you are making and add one new habit at a time. Use the weekly reflection checklist on your journey and make sure you evaluate at the end of each week so you notice how every implementation is providing more ease and more relief to your symptoms.

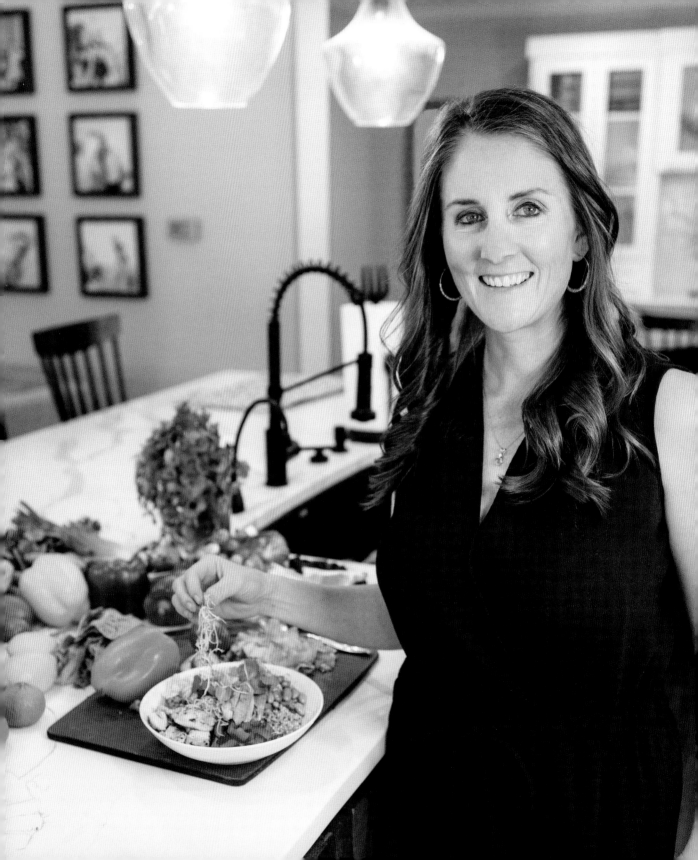

Understanding Your Symptoms

If you don't know why your symptoms are happening, its hard to know what to do in order to relieve them. Perhaps this is why you feel stuck. This section of the book will help you understand the symptoms you are experiencing and create an action plan for relief.

Whether it's painful gas, debilitating constipation or frequent diarrhea, no one should have to struggle with symptoms that impact their ability to live life to the fullest. In this chapter, we will discuss common digestive complaints, how to resolve them and how to prevent them from coming back.

Constipation

One of the most common complaints that I hear and see my clients struggling with is constipation. Constipation is defined as fewer than four bowel movements per week, but in my experience and opinion, you should be emptying your bowels every day. If not, you could be constipated. Constipation can be embarrassing, frustrating and uncomfortable, but if you experience these symptoms, you are in the right place. This chapter should help you identify the common causes of your constipation and what you can do about them.

In the next section, you will learn about the Bristol Stool Scale chart in more depth (stay tuned, the drawings are vivid), but your stool should be soft, easy to pass, and like a snake (also see Appendix G [page 161]). If that is not your experience and you are straining, forcing or pushing, then constipation is a concern.

Some of the top triggers for constipation include:

- Dehydration
- Stress
- Lack of fiber
- Too little or too much movement
- Grazing or snacking all day
- Lack of sleep
- Slow gut motility
- Travel
- Metabolic disorders
- Hormone imbalances
- Disorders that affect the brain and spine
- Medications (e.g., painkillers, antidepressants, non-steroidal anti-inflammatories [NSAIDs], iron pills, allergy medications)

In addition to the uncomfortable pain and bloating that you may experience due to constipation, if left unaddressed, it can lead to more serious complications like anal fissures, hemorrhoids, diverticulitis, fecal impaction, damage to the pelvic floor muscles, rectal prolapse and small intestinal bacterial overgrowth (SIBO). If you have suffered from any of these common complications, resolving your constipation is key to ensuring that these conditions do not return.

Typically, with severe constipation, diet alone will not resolve your constipation, which is why this book covers other methods to improve constipation beyond food. Many of my clients have gone to the doctor and been told that to resolve their constipation they needed to "drink more water and eat more fiber." They leave feeling frustrated and hopeless as a result, worrying that they will never find relief because they have "been there, done that." It is true that dehydration is one of the most common triggers for constipation, but in the section on hydration (page 36), I will explain to you why sometimes just drinking water is not enough. I hope that this chapter empowers you with tools beyond the typical "drink more water and eat more fiber" recommendation.

The goal is to equip you to be proactive about your digestion, even if you are out of your routine (e.g., travel, new work routine, at a friend's house for dinner, etc.).

Finding the correct "constipation cocktail" can be tricky, but here are some of the top things that you can do today to start improving your constipation:

- Drink 80–100 ounces (2.4–3 L) of water per day; add electrolytes if needed (see the hydration section on page 36 for more information on this)

- Avoid excess raw vegetables and fruits; try switching to very well-cooked fruits and veggies to improve digestion

- Avoid excess alcohol

- Try the "I Love You" massage (see page 34)

- Increase consumption of magnesium-rich foods (see Appendix B on page 153) or talk to your medical provider about using a magnesium supplement (ex: magnesium citrate)

- Stimulate the migrating motor complex by spacing your meals out every 3–4 hours

- Drink ginger tea in between meals (ginger helps your gut to contract and move food/waste through)

- Slowly add in prebiotic fiber (e.g., acacia fiber; partially hydrolyzed guar gum). Start with ½ teaspoon in week 1, increase to 1 teaspoon in week 2, increase to 2+ teaspoons in week 3

- Get regular exercise and incorporate gentle movement throughout the day

- Add in stress-reducing activities daily (ex: deep breathing, nature walks, laughter or yoga)

- Get 7–8 hours of sleep per night

- Avoid holding it or ignoring the urge to go

- Check your physical positioning on toilet (knees above hips; a Squatty Potty® can be useful for this)

If you're still constipated after implementing these habits, then it's important to consider your gut–brain connection, gut motility, your stress levels and your migrating motor complex. Each of these systems affects constipation. I go over all these systems in detail in later chapters, so stay tuned!

How to Know If You're Constipated:

- Log how often you have a bowel movement

- Note its characteristics

- Note whether you feel your bowel movement was complete

- After, you should feel happy and satisfied; you should not feel as though you have to strain, push or squeeze

- Track your Bristol Stool Scale number (see Appendix G on page 161)

Foods to include for constipation

Most plant foods contain a combination of different fibers, but some foods specifically help in aiding constipation. If you are constipated, try incorporating some of the foods listed below to help relieve your symptoms:

- Prunes (eat 3 prunes, 3 times per day or drink ½ cup [120 ml] of 100% prune juice)
- Kiwi (eat one to two whole kiwi fruits per day)
- Ground flaxseed (slowly work toward eating 3 tablespoons [25 g] per day)
- Chia seeds (slowly work toward 2 tablespoons [22 g] per day)
- Beans (consider sprouted or soaked beans for easier digestion)
- Oats (consider soaked or sprouted)
- Bananas
- Blackberries
- Pears
- Blueberries
- Grapes
- Peaches
- Figs
- Apples
- Citrus fruit
- Sweet potato
- Insulin-rich foods: asparagus, chicory, garlic, Jerusalem artichoke, leeks, oats, onions, soybeans
- Pectin-rich foods: citrus peels, apples, plums, gooseberries, cherries, apricots, carrots, beets, bananas, cabbage, dried peas, okra

Gas

Gas is another one of the common complaints that we see with our clients, and it is typically coupled with constipation, bloating and/or diarrhea. But first, let's normalize that everyone toots. The average person passes gas 20 times per day and 99 percent is odorless or pleasant. Gas should be easy to pass and odorless. It is also normal to have gas after eating certain foods, such as beans and cruciferous vegetables like Brussels sprouts, broccoli and cauliflower.

So, what happens if it isn't odorless or due to eating some of the foods mentioned above?

If your gas is sulfur smelling, it's important to consider your protein intake (high amounts of protein from meat can contribute to gas), your egg intake and/or your cruciferous vegetable intake.

If your gas is consistently smelly but not sulphury, the smell could indicate that there is damage to your microbiome or general gut bacterial imbalances (see page 23 for more about this).

If you have gas immediately after eating this can be a result of the gastro-colic reflex, which indicates that the colon is starting to move after eating to accommodate room for the new food. If you struggle with consistently smelly gas after eating make sure that you are practicing meal hygiene and calming your nervous system before eating to allow your digestive tract to be in "rest and digest" mode.

If your gas comes in clusters, the most common trigger for this is constipation. If it smells, it could be food intolerances (e.g., lactose intolerance). The main causes for stinky gas include lactose intolerance or sugar alcohol consumption (any non-nutritive sweetener ending in -ol [e.g., sorbitol], celiac disease and certain medications).

Regardless of what triggers your gas, here are some strategies and interventions that you can use to manage it while you are addressing what is truly causing it:

- Make sure you aren't constipated

- Eat fennel seeds or drink peppermint tea after eating

- Focus on sprouted foods and fewer raw veggies

- Decrease fiber consumption first, then work on reintroducing fiber slowly

- Focus on meal hygiene. Meal hygiene refers to the concept of how and when you eat. Before you even think about what you are eating, assess how you are eating. (See more about this on page 26)

- Avoid bubbly and carbonated drinks, drinking through straws and chewing gum

Diarrhea

Diarrhea is defined as loose watery stools three or more times per day. It can be acute, persistent or chronic. Common triggers for diarrhea include stress, nervous system dysregulation, foods or food additives (see below), lack of fiber, dehydration or a gut infection.

One of the most important messages that I want you to understand about diarrhea is that if it comes and goes, you might actually be constipated. If you go days without a bowel movement, then have diarrhea in between, you could have what is called "overflow diarrhea." This form of diarrhea is actually the most severe form of constipation. I want you to imagine filling your bathtub with water and then trying to drain it with the drain closed. Eventually the water will overflow. Even though you have 25 feet [7.6 m] of intestines and lots of storage room, it is possible to fill it up and run out of space if you are actually constipated and your bowels are unable to clear themselves. If this describes your diarrhea pattern, try tips for alleviating constipation, rather than diarrhea.

If you struggle with diarrhea, it is important to assess what is triggering it (e.g., food, environment, etc.) and track patterns if you can. It can be common that individuals will experience diarrhea in a pattern, for example, having loose stools every time they leave the house or every time they are on their way to work. If this is the case, working on regulating the nervous system and rewiring the brain to have positive associations with these circumstances is necessary (see the Nervous System Function/Neuroplasticity section on page 38 for more information).

If your diarrhea wakes you up in the middle of the night, it might be worth a visit to a gastrointestinal (GI) doctor to be evaluated for inflammatory bowel disease. Unless you have a food poisoning episode or the stomach flu (which typically passes quickly), your bowels should not wake you up in the middle of the night.

If you are struggling with diarrhea, adding fiber from food (and potentially supplementation) will be extremely helpful in resolving some of your symptoms.

Below are some foods that are helpful for binding the stool and improving diarrhea:

- Bananas

- Broccoli (start with ½ cup [35 g] of *cooked* broccoli [or less]) low and slow

- Brussels sprouts (start with ½ cup [80 g] of *cooked* Brussels sprouts [or less]) low and slow

- Apples

- Beans such as chickpeas (start low and go slow and try sprouted or canned; be sure to drain, rinse and drain again canned beans or lentils)

- Eggplant

- Okra
- Oranges
- Passion fruit
- Sunflower seeds
- Mashed turnips
- Cooked carrots
- Ground flaxseeds
- Lentils (start low and go slow or try sprouting them)
- Oats (can trial gluten free/sprouted if adding back)
- Oat bran
- Sweet potatoes
- Mangos
- Plums
- Berries
- Peaches
- Kiwi
- Figs

If needed, add fiber powder—acacia fiber or psyllium husk—to bulk up stool:

- **Acacia fiber:** start with ½ teaspoon twice a day, gradually increase your dose by ½ teaspoon each time of the day every 3–5 days until you reach the full dose of 2 teaspoons (10 g) total (divided doses) up to 3 tablespoons (45 g) total (divided doses)

- **Psyllium husk:** start with 1 teaspoon twice a day, gradually increase your dose by 1 teaspoon each time of the day every 3–5 days until you reach the full dose of 2 tablespoons (30 g) twice per day

Some common foods or food additives that can trigger a diarrhea episode:

- Alcohol: speeds up gut motility
- Caffeine (found in coffee; white, black and green tea; and large amounts of chocolate): speeds up gut motility
- Sugar alcohols like sorbitol, erythritol, mannitol, etc. (anything that ends in -ol, be sure to check labels)
- Artificial sweeteners like aspartame, sucralose, and saccharin, etc. (check labels)
- Greasy or fried foods (fried chicken, French fries, etc.)
- Dairy (try lactose-free dairy for 4 weeks to see if this improves your symptoms and to see if you might be lactose intolerant)

Action steps to improve diarrhea:

- Include stress management daily
  - Deep diaphragmatic breathing like the 4–7–8 relaxation breath (breathe in for 4 seconds, hold for 7 seconds, breathe out for 8 seconds, then repeat) or box breathing (breathe in for 4 seconds, hold for 4 seconds, breathe out for 4 seconds, hold for 4 seconds, then repeat)
  - Meditation (try using a guided app such as Calm® or Headspace®)
  - Focusing on neuroplasticity (see Appendix C [page 154])
  - Start your day with gratitude by writing down three specific things you are grateful for (e.g., I am grateful that I slept for 7 hours last night)
  - Vagus nerve stimulation (gargling, humming, ending showers [the last 60 seconds] in cold water) to improve the gut–brain connection
  - IBS hypnotherapy app (Nerva)
- Stay hydrated
- Try marshmallow root tea or passionflower tea to calm the stomach and soothe the intestines

Bloating

Bloating is a common complaint, but sometimes it can also be a normal reaction to food. It's important to understand the difference.

What Is Normal?

The average person passes gas 20 times per day, but for the most part it is odorless air.

There are certain foods that are considered "gas forming" and therefore can contribute to the bloat that you might experience outside of the norm. Some foods that can contribute to bloating include broccoli, cauliflower, Brussels sprouts, beans, lentils and chickpeas. If you commonly bloat after eating these foods, you're not alone. The bloating should subside after a few hours and if it does, that is normal. It can also be normal to bloat after eating a larger plate of vegetables (even ones not listed above). If you consume large amounts of raw fiber at the same time, expect that your stomach might feel a little bloated.

What Is Not Normal?

If your bloating has become painful, chronic and persistent, it is likely not normal. Oftentimes our clients will state that they feel "full of hot air" or "feel 6 months pregnant by the end of the day." If you experience these symptoms, you are not alone. Identifying patterns in your bloating can help you identify why you're bloated in the first place.

The cause of the bloating matters, so after you have identified the cause, below are some action steps that you can take to improve your bloating and find relief:

- Address constipation
- Drink plenty of water (80–100 ounces [2.4–3 L] per day)
- Avoid known triggers for bloating
  - Bubbly water
  - Eating too quickly (make your meals last 20 minutes)
  - Straws
  - Chewing gum
  - Sucking on candy
- Relax: Allow your body to get into rest/digest mode before eating (Tip: Try humming "Happy Birthday" to yourself twice before eating)
- Stimulate migrating motor complex by spacing out meals by 3–4 hours
- Drink ginger tea between meals to help with gut motility and constipation

If you are waking up bloated	→ Take a look at your gut motility and make sure that you are not constipated
If you are bloating within an hour of eating	→ Take a look at digestive insufficiencies and evaluate if you need enzymes or stomach acid support
If you're getting progressively more bloated toward the end of the day	→ You could potentially have dysbiosis (see page 23)

Acid Reflux

It's not uncommon for those who struggle with bloat and constipation to also struggle with acid reflux. Acid reflux can be debilitating, frustrating and uncomfortable. Conventionally, one of the most prescribed medications in the world is acid reflux medication. Unfortunately, these medications can cause more issues downstream and shouldn't be relied upon for long term relief. Proton pump inhibitors (PPIs) and acid reflux medications decrease the amount of stomach acid and as a result can slow down gut motility, impact gut bacterial balance and impair nutrient absorption. For many individuals, the cause of their acid reflux is actually low, not high, stomach acid, so taking medication to further decrease stomach acid could potentially be making the problem worse.

We need adequate stomach acid to:

- Denature proteins and activate the enzyme pepsin, which further digests protein

- Prevent the overgrowth of "bad" or dysbiotic bacteria

- Absorb vitamins like B_{12}

- Trigger the release of cholecystokinin (CCK), which stimulates the release of bile from the gallbladder

If you are struggling with acid reflux here are some common triggers to keep in mind:

- Too little stomach acid (can mimic symptoms of high stomach acid)

- Stress (probably the most common trigger I see)

- Zinc and magnesium deficiency (needed to produce stomach acid)

- Poor meal hygiene (see more on this below, and in later chapters)

- *H. pylori* infections

To start improving your acid reflux, here are some important action steps you can take:

- **Practice proper meal hygiene:** Meal hygiene refers to the concept of how and when you eat. Before you even think about what you are eating, assess how you are eating. Taking the time to chew your food and eat slowly is a game changer for digestion.

- **Don't undereat:** When you are undereating you are creating more stress on the body and as a result, the stomach produces less acid. It becomes a vicious cycle both physiologically and with symptoms.

- **Engage in 5 to 15 minutes of stress management:** Can you sense a theme here? Stress impacts stomach acid production and can contribute to deficiencies in nutrients needed to produce stomach acid (like sodium and magnesium). Taking 5 minutes a day to get outside or do something that relieves stress makes a big difference.

- Assess if certain foods could be contributing and limit if needed until you have been able to resolve the acid reflux. Some common triggers for acid reflux symptoms include:

  - Fried, greasy foods

  - Chocolate

  - Coffee

  - Mint (like peppermint)

  - Alcohol

  - Onions

  - Citrus fruits and juices (lemon, orange, grapefruit, etc.)

  - Tomatoes and tomato products

  - Spicy foods (pepper, curry, etc.)

  - Carbonated drinks (sodas, waters, beer, etc.)

- **Try to avoid eating immediately before bed:** The stomach needs time to empty, so give yourself adequate time between your last meal and bedtime to decrease acid reflux at bedtime.

- **Consider taking a magnesium supplement to open your lower pyloric valve and empty the stomach:** 200 to 400 mg of magnesium can be helpful in allowing your stomach contents to empty and decrease acid reflux symptoms.

- **Try aloe juice for unwanted symptoms:** Pure aloe juice found at a local health food store can be super soothing to the digestive tract; 2 to 4 ounces (60 to 120 ml) of aloe juice in water, tea or a smoothie is a great symptom relief tool.

- Use slippery elm tea when you experience reflux (in either tea or capsule form). Purchase at your local health food store or online at Mountain Rose Herbs®.

- Use deglycerized licorice before meals.

- Consider weaning off of your PPI (e.g., omeprazole); talk with your medical provider.

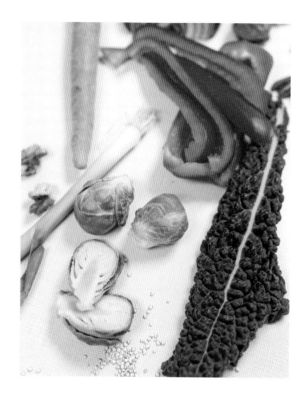

What Your Poop Says About Your Symptoms

The color, shape, size and texture of your poop says a lot about what is going on in your body. I know, it can be uncomfortable to talk about poop, but we are all friends here, and everyone poops! Knowing your poop patterns can empower you to address them.

The Bristol Stool Scale (see Appendix G on page 161)

The Bristol Stool Scale is a measurement tool that you can utilize to see how things are going. The goal is for your stool to look like a snake, be soft, and also be easy to pass. In fact, having a bowel movement should feel effortless. It is normal to have one to three bowel movements per day, and there should be no food in your stool (other than corn and quinoa). Going to the bathroom three times a day doesn't necessarily mean that your digestion is better. Whether you go to the bathroom one or three times a day, the most important piece is that you are completely emptying your bowels daily. For some individuals, it will be possible to do this in one bowel movement, and others it may take three movements. It could just mean that your gut is more efficient at clearing out stool all at once. The goal is that you should feel satisfied, content and like there was nothing left.

If your stool is between a 1 and 3 on the Bristol Stool Scale you are likely constipated. If it is between a 5 and 7 then you are experiencing diarrhea. Using this scale can help you to navigate what interventions to utilize when addressing your symptoms.

The Color of Your Stool

Your stool should be brown. When it is not, it's important to take note and determine next steps. Below are some deviations and explanations for possible causes:

- **Pale:** If your stool is pale, it could be due to a blockage in the liver or bile duct. You may need pancreatic, gallbladder or stomach acid support.

- **Green:** If your stool is green, it could be due to a gut infection, antibiotics or eating a lot of leafy greens.

- **Red:** If your stool is red, make sure it is not blood. If it is not, it could be due to eating beets.

- **Yellow:** If your stool is yellow, it is important to determine if you need pancreatic support.

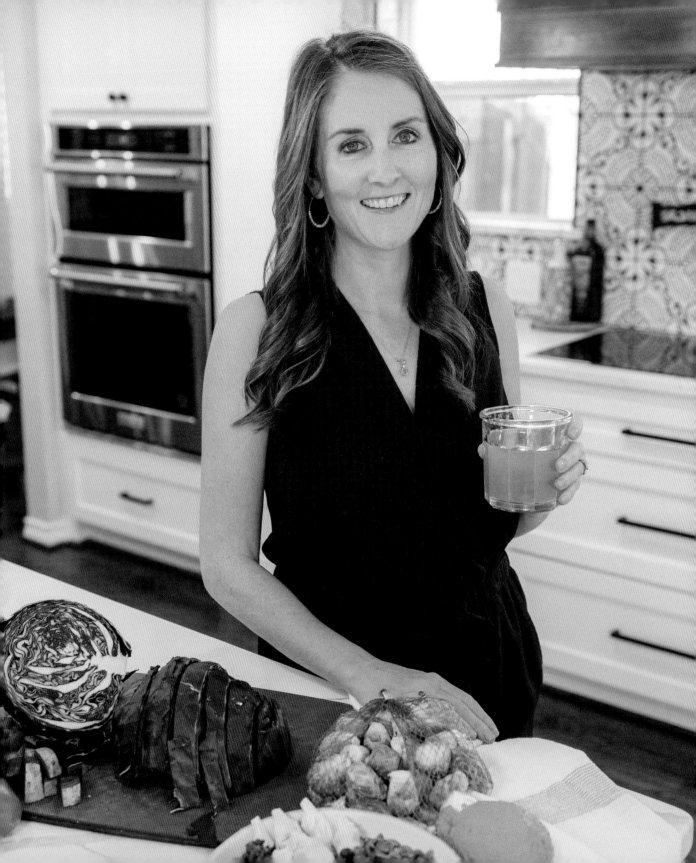

Gut Dysbiosis

What Is "the Gut"?

The gut refers to the entire digestive tract starting from the mouth and ending at your anus. The mouth contains salivary glands that release saliva and when food enters your mouth, the amount of saliva that you produce increases to help lubricate food and start breaking it down. As you have already learned, your gut is full of bacteria. In fact, you have more bacteria than you do human cells! Everyone has their own unique gut microbiota makeup and there is not a "perfect" makeup of gut bacteria (that we know of yet). Your gut microbiota is as unique as your fingerprint.

Gut dysbiosis is a broad term describing what happens when your bacteria are imbalanced. Your gut is full of colonies of bacteria. Most of these bacteria have a positive effect on your health and contribute to your body's natural processes and systems. For example, the healthy bacteria in your gut, like the lactobacillus and bifidobacterium, improve your digestive symptoms. Dysbiosis occurs when these colonies of helpful and beneficial bacteria get out of balance or decrease in quantity. Any interruption in the balance of your gut microbiota can cause dysbiosis. For example, a dietary change that reduces your fiber intake, taking antibiotics, poor dental hygiene, and high levels of stress. You will always have "bad" or unwanted bacteria in your gut.

Bacterial balance in your gut is important not only for the state of your gut but also for the health of your brain, metabolism, cardiovascular health and other body systems. Sleep patterns, exercise, antibiotic exposure, nutrition, socioeconomic status, education, genetics, medical care and environment can all have an impact on your gut bacteria, so focusing on nutrition is just one piece of the puzzle.

Diversity and the stability of the microbes you have in your gut are key indicators of health and promote disease prevention and metabolism improvement. As a result of gut dysbiosis, you may experience symptoms such as diarrhea, cramping, constipation, bloating or indigestion.

The other important thing you want to know about your gut microbes is that they actually help you digest fiber. As you read further into this book, you will discover the amazing impact that fiber has on your gut health and how eating fiber is one of the keys to improving your symptoms.

A controversial question in the gut health world is: Do we "starve" or "kill" the "bad" bacteria so that the good can take over? Or: How do we include fiber without the symptoms and increase the beneficial gut bacteria? When addressing dysbiosis, we need to have the "good guys" around so that they can do the heavy lifting for you. Instead of just focusing on "killing" your "bad guys" (ex: "starving the bacteria by not eating any fiber, carbs or foods that cause symptoms) you need to build up an army of "good guys" to defend you. I cannot tell you how many times we have worked with clients who have seen other practitioners and taken loads of herbs, antibiotics and supplements to "kill" their "bad" bacteria, but there was never a discussion of how to foster a healthy gut environment to allow the "good gut bugs" to flourish through diet and lifestyle. If you have just focused on "killing" in the past, then this book is for you. If you implement strategies to foster a healthy environment for your "good" bacteria to thrive and flourish, you can make lasting changes in your gut health. Your "no sugar" and "low carb" diet is starving your gut bacteria and creating a vicious cycle of symptoms for you.

When you have lower levels of beneficial bacteria in your gut, eating fiber can induce unwanted symptoms like bloating/distention, cramping and constipation, but keep in mind that your gut is a muscle. Go low and slow reintroducing rich fiber sources (even 1 tablespoon at a time) and you will reap the rewards of fueling your beneficial gut bacteria and ultimately change the ecosystem of your gut for the better. The number one thing you can do for your gut health is get your "good" bacteria on board by including a diverse variety of fiber sources as well as focusing on all the tips I suggest in the Beyond Diet section (see page 25).

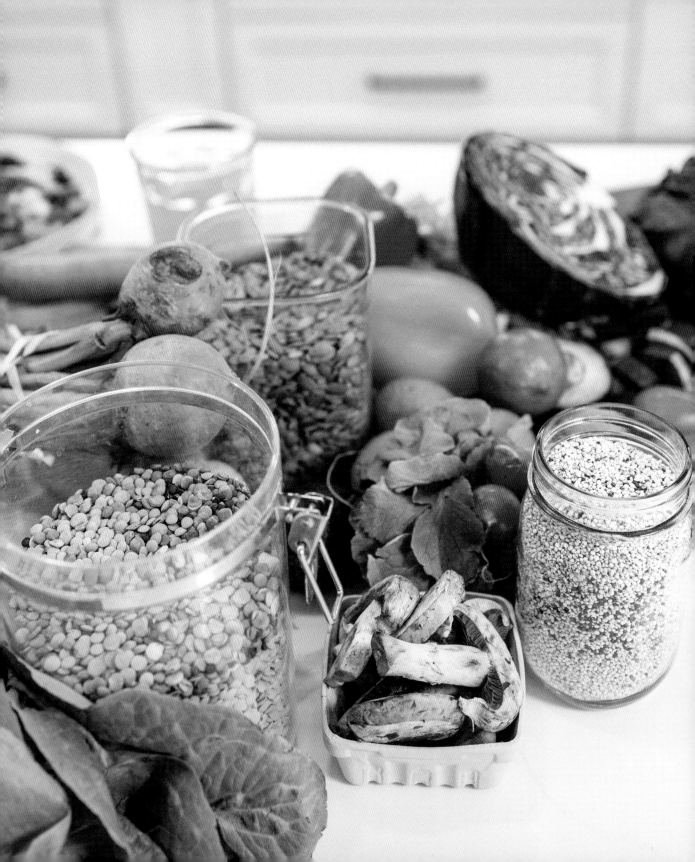

How You're Eating

When you experience digestive distress, it's easy to quickly think it is related to something you ate—but what if it actually isn't? What if your symptoms were more related to how you ate or your environment versus the food itself? We would be missing some very critical pieces of digestion if we only discussed food and didn't place an emphasis on how you are eating.

My clients generally come to me assuming that food is the source of all their digestive troubles. While food choices certainly play a role for many people, there are loads of other factors that affect digestion—and have nothing to do with the food itself. This section describes some basic mechanics of digestion and offers a list of ways to improve your gut health without changing anything about your diet.

Beyond Diet: Setting the Stage for Proper Digestion

As a dietitian, one of the first questions I am often asked is "What do I eat for a healthy gut?" But, before we even talk about what to eat for any type of digestive struggle, we must first address the foundational principles of gut health (which surprisingly have nothing to do with food!).

How you eat, what you think and how you approach your meal can move the needle on your digestive symptoms way more than you might think.

Understanding Digestion

First, let's break down how digestion works. I want you to think about a time when you were walking down the street, smelled your favorite pastry and started salivating. You probably weren't hungry until you actually smelled the pastry.

This process is the first phase of digestion—before food ever even enters your mouth there are communication pathways in your body that are turned on when you start to salivate. Your saliva stimulates the stomach, liver, gallbladder and pancreas, all of which are involved in digestion, to start secreting enzymes and acid for digestion.

So now, you decide to go into the bakery and purchase the pastry and you take a bite of the delicious, fluffy dough. You chew it up and, because of the steps listed above, your stomach is ready for digestion the second that the pastry enters your mouth. Your liver, gallbladder and pancreas all play a role in digesting the carbohydrates, proteins and fats found in this pastry so they can hand it off to the small intestine where most of your nutrients are absorbed.

This process can be disrupted by many different factors and can impact how the body (and the gut) digest and absorb food.

Have you ever had an experience where you drove somewhere and when you arrived you didn't remember how you even got there? If your brain is running on autopilot while eating, the actual process of digestion will not be as effective. We do this all the time. We eat while we work, while we drive, while we are watching TV or while our brain is in a completely different space. When we do this, we are less likely to chew and mechanically break down our food so that it can be digested well.

Your stomach acid and digestive enzymes are responsible for breaking food down once they enter your stomach, but you are responsible for breaking your food down (via chewing) before that happens. There's no perfect way to do this, but what you need to know is that food should be the consistency of applesauce before you swallow.

Your eating experience should not be rushed. If possible, try to sit at the table, with no distractions, for 15 to 20 minutes. I promise, you won't regret it!

The process of eating should be as intentional as possible, and should also be an opportunity for your body to rest and digest. The societal pressure of working with no breaks in the day or being able to say "I didn't even have time for lunch" has got to go. When you prioritize these first steps of digestion, everything else downstream functions better.

Thousands of our clients have made these changes and found that the simple act of reconnecting around the table with their families and friends has not only improved their digestion, but decreased their stress because it has provided a natural break in the day that they begin to look forward to.

Meal Hygiene

The process that I just described is called meal hygiene. Meal hygiene is one of the most effective (and free!) ways that you can improve your digestion. And it all happens before you even lift your fork.

Your homework: For one meal a day, devote time to sitting down, taking the time to eat a meal and chewing your food. Log how you feel after eating and what changes you notice in your body. I think you'll be surprised.

Here are some things that you can think about when you are implementing the process of meal hygiene:

- Before taking a bite, notice what you smell

- Before taking a bite, take three deep breaths (my favorite breathing exercise is called 4–7–8 breathing: breathe in for 4, hold for 7 and out for 8)

- After taking your first bite, notice the different flavors of the food

- Set your fork down in between bites and really chew your food to applesauce consistency

- When possible, eat with others

- After you are finished eating, try to sit and linger over conversation for a few minutes

Pro Tip: The amount of saliva you release is controlled by your nervous system. A certain amount of saliva is normally present, but even the thought, sight or smell of food can stimulate more saliva (the cephalic phase of digestion). When the body is stressed, saliva production decreases, which further emphasizes the importance of meal hygiene and stress management when focusing on gut health.

The tongue helps to push food through to the back of the mouth and the esophagus further produces mucus to help lubricate food and make swallowing easier. If the esophageal muscles are weak, swallowing becomes harder.

When you eat and chew food, it passes through your esophagus, into your stomach and then into the small intestine. Shortly after food enters your stomach, the muscles of the stomach start to contract, which helps the stomach contents mix with the gastric juices to improve digestion. After the stomach has adequately digested food, it pushes small amounts into the small intestine. For this process to work, you must be able to swallow, produce adequate stomach acid and adequate digestive enzymes.

Another key contributor to this process is the nervous system. As you learned in the meal hygiene section (page 26), before you even begin eating, your brain is sending signals to your digestive tract to prepare it for digestion. If the nervous system is stressed or dysregulated, this process can be disrupted.

The small intestine has three sections: the duodenum, the jejunum and the ileum. These three sections are critically important for nutrient absorption and where food is digested and absorbed into the bloodstream. The villi, which are small finger-like projections with blood vessels inside of the intestinal wall, optimize absorption and allow nutrients released by digestion to enter the blood.

After food passes through the last part of the ileum in the small intestine, it enters the large intestine, otherwise known as the colon. The large intestine is much smaller in size compared to the small intestine, which is approximately 25 feet (7.6 m) long. The large intestine houses the gut microbiota, which is made up of trillions of cells and houses the largest population of bacteria, viruses and fungi in the body (more on this later). When chime (digested food) has been in the large intestine for 3 to 10 hours, it becomes semi-solid and the remnants become stools. The movements in the large intestine (peristalsis) help to move the chime and stool toward the rectum. The large intestine absorbs water and contains food that has not been digested, such as fiber. After the fiber is digested and water is absorbed, the waste makes its way toward the rectum, where stool is stored until it is ready to be pushed out through the back passage, otherwise known as the anus. The anus is a muscular opening that is usually closed, unless stool is passing through.

The entire process of digestion breaks food down into its most basic parts so that it can be absorbed, utilized and transported throughout the body.

What Does the Gut Do?

The gut processes food throughout the entire digestive process until it is either absorbed or passed as stool. The process of digestion starts well before food ever enters the mouth or it is mechanically broken down by chewing.

Certain chemicals produced in the stomach (like hydrochloric acid) help with digestion and food breakdown and most of the nutrients from food are absorbed in the large intestine. In addition to hydrochloric acid, there are specific enzymes involved in the chemical breakdown of food that help the body get adequate nutrition from food. Acid and enzymes also help to move food through your digestive tract so that you can eliminate it. Anything that cannot be digested—waste substances, bacteria, germs or undigested food—are then eliminated as stool.

Our GI tracts are intimately linked to our overall health and well-being. Home to more than 100 trillion microorganisms, collectively known as the "gut microbiota," its primary function is digestion, absorption of nutrients and the excretion of waste. In addition to these functions, the GI tract also has a major influence on the development and function of the immune system as well as on how the gut and the brain communicate with each other.

- 70% to 80% of the body's immune cells are in the gut

- There are 100 million neurons located in the gut that impact neurotransmitter production (mood) and regulate fullness, pain and hunger

- 95% of the body's serotonin (the hormone that helps you feel calm) is in your gut

- It might be surprising, but you actually have more bacteria on and in your body than you do human cells!

The Migrating Motor Complex

Did you know that your gut has its own cleanup crew? Oftentimes this clean-up crew doesn't show up because we are working late (aka eating small snacks, not large meals). When you are able to space your meals out every 3 to 4 hours your migrating motor complex crew shows up to sweep out the intestines, therefore relieving bloat and constipation. One of the most helpful shifts you can make to improve your digestion is moving from snacking all day long to eating well-balanced, spaced-out meals and giving your gut time to "rest and digest" in between.

A few key things to consider:

- Be sure to eat enough at meals so that you are satisfied for 3 to 4 hours (see the section on building a gut-happy plate on page 51)

- Hunger trumps all, so if you do get hungry between meals, it is more important to eat and respond to your hunger cues than abide by the clock

- This shift could take some time (maybe even months!); work on spacing out one meal at a time instead of doing this all at once since your blood sugar and your body need time to adapt

The Enteric Nervous System

The enteric nervous system (ENS), otherwise known as your second brain, oversees the functions of the GI tract and is the nervous system of the GI tract. It has more than 100 million neurons, which is more neurons than anywhere else in the body. The ENS is connected to the gut through the vagus nerve and assists with moving smooth muscles, and secreting neurotransmitters and various peptides.

The ENS also contains the gut microbiota, which helps to make neurotransmitters and vitamins, supports the immune system and modulates intestinal permeability (what you may have heard of as a "leaky gut"). The ENS also makes short chain fatty acids (more on this later), which are important for memory, mood and inflammation.

The Gut–Brain Connection

The gut and the brain are connected and communicate directly with each other, so what is going on in the gut is also going on in the brain. Oftentimes we tell our clients an anxious mind = an anxious gut. When they can connect the emotions they are feeling to the gut symptoms they are having, it can be incredibly empowering for navigating difficult symptoms. The central nervous system and the organs of the GI tract communicate through the largest cranial nerve in the body, known as the vagus nerve. The bacteria in the gut impact the communication up to the brain via the vagus nerve, and vice versa. The more bacterial diversity you have in your gut, the happier your brain.

When the nervous system is functioning in a fight-or-flight response the following things happen:

- Pupils dilate

- Salivation is inhibited

- Heart rate increases

- Airways relax

- Stomach activity is inhibited

- Gallbladder activity is inhibited

- Glucose is released to increase blood sugar

- Intestinal activity is halted

These responses greatly impact how the body can digest and absorb food, which is why it is so important to think about how your nervous system is responding to situations, to food and to your environment.

When your nervous system is in a "rest and digest" state the following functions occur:

- Saliva production is stimulated
- Heartbeat slows
- Airways constrict
- Stomach activity is promoted
- Glucose is not released
- Gallbladder secretions increase
- Intestinal activity resumes

Activating the "rest and digest" system in the body is critical for proper digestion and could be one of the reasons so many people experience digestive symptoms. In our busy culture, we are often way too stressed, rarely leaving time for relaxation, fun and enjoyment. Simply focusing on getting the body into a "rest and digest" state is fundamental to healthy digestion, and one way you can do this is by activating the vagus nerve.

Activating the Vagus Nerve

Activating the vagus nerve to help increase communication to the gut from the brain is a key component of gut health. When you activate the vagus nerve (the superhighway between the gut and the brain), you are promoting digestion, activating the parasympathetic nervous system and improving gut motility. Some of the simple daily activities that you can do to promote vagus nerve stimulation include:

- Gargling with water (2–3 minutes per day). Instructions: Pour yourself a glass of water and gargle for as long as you can until you need to take a breath. When you need to take a breath, spit out the water, take a breath, then take another sip and continue. Repeat until the glass is finished.

Note about gargling: If you gargle for 25 seconds, this is your "baseline" time. Work your way up to 2 to 3 minutes (breaths included). Do 25 seconds twice daily for 1 week. Then, re-time yourself the following week. If you now can tolerate 35 seconds of gargling, this is your new baseline time and you should gargle 35 seconds twice daily for the next week. Slowly build up tolerance until you can gargle for 2 to 3 minutes (you can take breaks to breathe)

- Humming "Happy Birthday" twice before eating your meal
- Singing at a high octave (think opera style!)
- Turning the shower on cold for 30–60 seconds at the end
- Diaphragmatic breathing

The gut and the brain are always communicating, but the connection can be disrupted by present and even past circumstances. Past trauma; route of birth (C-section or vaginal delivery); brain injuries; gut dysbiosis and pathogens; inflammation; and medications like antibiotics, PPIs and NSAIDS can impact how well the gut communicates with the brain. Your gut bacterial diversity is also important for gut–brain communication, so anything that disturbs the abundance of bacteria in the gut is going to impact how well this communication pathway functions (see the Dysbiosis section on page 23 for more information). Additionally, food poisoning, low short chain fatty acid production (from lack of fiber in the diet and diversity of gut microbes) and current stress can impact this connection.

The gut is ever changing and evolving, so although there are factors that can contribute to the overall diversity of the gut and gut composition; it is adaptable given the proper stimulus (dietary diversity, adequate stress management, etc.).

To address the gut–brain connection and optimize the vagus nerve connection, it is important to focus on the following in your diet: tons of fibrous diversity, omega-3 fatty acids from salmon and other fatty fish, prebiotic fiber and probiotics. See the Gut-Happy Plate section on page 51 for more information.

Gut Motility

Another important aspect of the gut–brain connection is how this system impacts the movement of the gut muscle. Motility is the movement of food and waste through your intestines. Ideally, after you eat a meal the food should be excreted within 12 to 24 hours. Unfortunately for those with IBS and other digestive issues, it can often be much longer (or sometimes shorter) than this. When you have a bowel movement, you should feel relieved afterward, and you should feel like there is nothing left. When the vagus nerve connection is weak from stress, trauma, food poisoning or any of the other factors listed above, it can impact the speed at which food moves through your system.

The migrating motor complex, the vagus nerve and your intestinal muscles (both small and large intestine) are all key components of this system. One of the reasons you might feel bloated, regardless of what you eat, or why you might wake up bloated could be slow gut motility. Thankfully, there are many things that you can do to improve the motility of your gut:

- Balance your blood sugar (see The Gut-Happy Plate section on page 51)
- Activate your vagus nerve through gargling, humming, singing or cold showers
- Decrease your stress and incorporate stress management day to day
- Practice deep, slow breathing
- Get adequate sleep every night
- Drink ginger tea between meals (ginger stimulates the gut muscles to contract)

- If you have had food poisoning, you can take a lions mane mushroom supplement OR consume lions mane mushrooms to help repair the nerve damage that results from food poisoning. If you are taking a capsule, look for a supplement that contains the fruiting body and is approx 1000mg.

Lifestyle Modifications for Gut Health

Stress and the Gut–Brain Connection

Stress is a repeat offender when it comes to disrupting digestion. Why? Historically, our bodies have relied on our nervous system's ability to respond to stress to survive. This is the "fight-or-flight" response that evolved to help us fend off or outrun predators. Unfortunately, when your body experiences any sort of stress, it can't distinguish between "I'm worried about being late to the dentist" or "I see a bear that might eat me." It only recognizes stress and responds accordingly.

How Does Stress Response Affect Digestion?

When your body experiences stress, it shifts resources away from non-essential functions like digestion to fuel your muscles and prepare your body to attack a predator or run away (i.e., fight or flight). Your gut secretes fewer digestive enzymes and less stomach acid, gut motility slows and essential nutrients are shuttled off to your muscles. Magnesium and potassium are two key players here. Both are critical for digestion and gut motility. When your body experiences stress, magnesium in your body that might otherwise be used for smooth digestion is re-prioritized to your muscles; your body also uses that magnesium and potassium at a higher rate when under a state of stress, which leads to a more rapid depletion of minerals.

Assess Your Stress

People commonly identify the stressors in their life as only coming from big things like jobs, relationships, child care or schooling. But stress can come in many forms, and it's the cumulative effect that matters. Subtler sources of stress include:

- Fear of food
- Negative food mindset (see below)
- Overexercising
- Lack of recovery after exercise
- Undereating in response to digestive discomfort or fear of food
- Lack of sleep and rest
- Dehydration
- Mineral and nutrient deficiencies (Magnesium, potassium, sodium, vitamin C and vitamin D are common ones)
- Lack of fun and enjoyment in life
- Hormone imbalances

Think of your stress as a threshold: a series of small stresses in your day can add up to have the effect of one big stress in your body without you even realizing it.

Stress Management

Managing your stress can have a *huge* impact on digestion. Just like a series of small stressors can add up throughout the day, so can a series of small stress-management steps. Taking a few moments to calm your nervous system helps reduce the overall amount of stress your body is experiencing and preserves important resources for your digestion. Committing to a regular practice of stress management also helps the body learn to calm its own nervous system, which contributes to overall lower stress over time. It's a win–win!

To help your body learn to calm its stress response, incorporate some of these stress-management strategies into your daily routine:

- Get outside in the sun for 10 minutes a day
- Call a friend
- Take an Epsom salt bath
- Listen to relaxing music
- Laugh
- Write in a gratitude journal

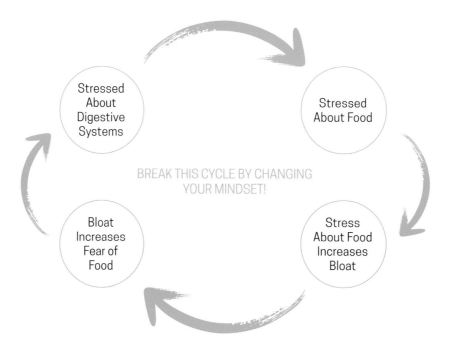

BREAK THIS CYCLE BY CHANGING YOUR MINDSET!

Stressed About Digestive Systems

Stressed About Food

Stress About Food Increases Bloat

Bloat Increases Fear of Food

Food Mindset

The way you think about food can trigger a stress response that directly affects digestion. By worrying that a food is going to cause bloating, you trigger your body's fight-or-flight response, almost guaranteeing that your body will have a negative digestive response, regardless of what you eat. It's a self-fulfilling prophecy in particularly cruel form. But here's the good news: by changing the way you think about food, you can improve the way your body digests it.

How to Change Your Food Mindset

Instead of seeing food as the cause of your digestive problems, it's important that you see food as a *tool* to help your digestion improve. This reframing is crucial in changing your food mindset, but it can take some time to embrace. Luckily, there are lots of little things in your control every time you eat. Focusing on these elements will help you gradually work toward embracing a food-as-nourishment mindset. To improve your symptoms, you will need to challenge your mindset about food and break the vicious cycle.

Step 1: Remember that your gut is a trainable muscle

The first step in changing your food mindset is challenging your belief that a particular food is problematic. Yes, it's possible that a food that's caused digestive distress in the past may cause it again in the future. But the gut is a muscle that can be trained over time to tolerate foods. Just because something caused a negative reaction in the past doesn't mean that it always will. Instead of viewing foods as "OK to eat" or "not OK to eat," work toward viewing every food as a means of training your gut.

Example:

Negative food mindset: "The last time I had garlic, it made me super bloated."

Challenge this mindset by asking:

- Have I ever had a positive digestive experience with garlic?

- How much garlic did I use last time? How could I reduce that volume of garlic in my current meal? For example, if you used a whole clove of garlic in a recipe, use a quarter clove.

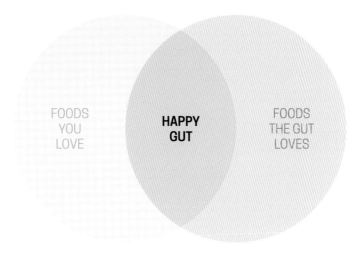

FOODS YOU LOVE

HAPPY GUT

FOODS THE GUT LOVES

Food-as-nourishment mindset: "I'm choosing to use a small amount of garlic in this meal to help train my gut to tolerate it. My gut is a muscle that can be trained and I hold the power to improve my digestion without restricting foods."

Step 2: Practice good meal hygiene

In addition to changing how you think about your food choices, you can also change your food mindset by focusing on the environment you create when you eat. Think of the following factors in your mealtime environment as "meal hygiene":

- **How quickly you're eating.** Eating a full meal should take about 20 minutes.

- **How well you're chewing your food.** You should chew each bite to the consistency of applesauce before swallowing.

- **Where you're eating.** Aim to eat in the same place each time you eat at home or work. Try to find a table and comfortable chair and use a place setting. Using a consistent routine helps cue your brain that it's time to eat and stimulates healthy digestion.

- **Who you're eating with.** How do your mealtime partners affect the pace of your eating? Do they bring you stress? Choose meal-mates who help you eat at a slow pace and in a relaxed state of mind.

- **Aesthetics.** What else helps you relax? Consider chill tunes, calming candles and soft lighting. Your standard for hosting a romantic date should be how you treat every meal for yourself.

The ability to control meal hygiene is also a valuable tool for those times when you don't have control over what you're eating. The next time you show up for a meal with a pre-set menu, focus on all the elements of the dining experience you *can* control rather than immediately assuming you'll have a bad digestive result. For more on the science behind this, see the Meal Hygiene section on page 26.

Movement

The gut is a muscle. Like any other muscle in the body, the gut needs exercise, making movement a valuable tool for tackling digestive issues. But just like other muscles, it's possible to overexercise the gut, so it's important to be mindful of how much you're moving. Too much exercise can also rob the body of energy needed to support digestion, because there's an energy cost required for your body to prioritize a bowel movement.

Gut-Friendly Movement

Any movement can stimulate the gut, but gentle movement is the most effective for stimulating healthy digestion. Activities like yoga, Pilates, light stretching and walking help your gut move without triggering a fight-or-flight response (see the Stress and the Gut-Brain Connection section on page 30 for more on this). You might love daily high-intensity interval training (HIIT) workouts, but it's possible that your exercise routine is making your digestive issues worse. Look for ways to incorporate more gentle movement into your exercise routine—you can always return to more strenuous activities when your gut is healthier.

Movement for Constipation

If you're experiencing constipation, develop a morning routine that includes gentle movement. You can also move your gut by practicing the "I Love You" massage twice daily. This massage, illustrated below, provides direct stimulation to your gut to help strengthen the muscle.

("I") Start on the left side of your body by the left side of your ribcage, pulse down toward the left hip bone for 15 seconds, gently massaging the colon.

(Upside down "L") Start at the right ribcage, move toward the left ribcage and down to the left hip for 20–30 seconds.

(Upside down "U") Start at the right hip and massage toward the right ribcage, then to the left ribcage to the left hip for 45 seconds.

Repeat this seuqence for a couple minutes morning and evening before going to sleep and after waking up to relieve gas and bloating.

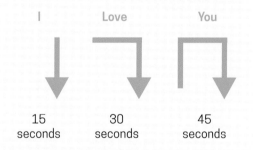

I	Love	You
15 seconds	30 seconds	45 seconds

Movement for Diarrhea

I know, I know, it seems like the last thing you'd want for diarrhea is more movement. Having chronic diarrhea doesn't mean you have to avoid exercise altogether, but it does mean you want to be thoughtful in the exercises you choose. Diarrhea is often a stress response, so focus on exercise that minimizes a stress response and minimizes strain on your pelvic floor—think low heart rate and low impact. Activities like yoga, Pilates, walking and gentle stretching all fit into this category.

Tips for managing diarrhea and exercise

If you typically experience diarrhea onset while exercising:

- Avoid caffeine before exercise and anything that will stimulate bowels

- Train your gut to tolerate a wider variety of foods and a higher volume of food over time by starting with easy-to-digest foods like bananas or toast, then gradually introducing new foods in small amounts before increasing the quantity

- Make sure that you stay hydrated and prioritize electrolytes and minerals in your water if you are having frequent bathroom trips

Sleep

The nervous system has two main functions: preparing you to fight or flee a predator and helping you rest and absorb the nutrients you've eaten that day. Your sympathetic nervous system controls your fight-or-flight response; your parasympathetic response controls the "rest-and-digest" functions. Our bodies are designed to have a lengthy amount of time to recover and digest. Unfortunately, modern culture doesn't encourage a lifestyle that prioritizes sleep. Most people need 7 to 8 hours of sleep every night but don't consistently get this amount.

How to Increase the Duration and Quality of Your Sleep

First, be aware of choices you make throughout the day that might be interfering with your sleep. Caffeine too late in the day, too much stimulation in the evening and waking up early to work out could all be adding stress and reducing your sleep. Your blood sugar balance also affects your sleep. If your blood sugar is dropping too low in the middle of the night, this could be the cause of frequent wake-ups (especially if this is happening every 2 to 3 hours). If you struggle with frequent wake-ups, prioritize your blood sugar balance throughout the day and consider consuming a balanced snack before bed. For more information on how to balance your blood sugar, see the Blood-Sugar Balance section on page 52.

To increase your sleep, try starting your nighttime routine 15 minutes earlier to accommodate an earlier bedtime.

Circadian Rhythm

Your circadian rhythm is very important for overall digestive health. Your body wants to be awake when it's light and asleep when it's dark; if you try to mirror the sun's pattern, it can be helpful for both your adrenal and digestive health. When you are asleep, your gut is actually "resting and digesting," which requires uninterrupted, deep, rest. The motto of "I will sleep when I am dead" is not doing your digestion any favors. Trust me, I've "been there, done that." If you focus on prioritizing sleep, you will see the payoff in symptoms, energy, productivity and mood just like our clients do.

If you work a shift job where you cannot follow this pattern, consider using a happy light while awake during night hours and try to sleep in a blacked-out room. Investing in blackout shades to mimic the dark can be very worthwhile. In addition, focus on what you *can* do (all the other tips in this book!) versus what you *can't* do.

Hydration

Whether you experience constipation or diarrhea, dehydration is one of the top triggers I see most commonly across all clients. Water is needed for many essential functions in the body, including your digestion. After all, the colon is a muscle; just like any other muscle in your body, it needs to be hydrated to work efficiently! Most individuals are consuming too much caffeine and/or too little water to adequately hydrate the colon and will experience negative side effects including decreased focus, decreased energy, increased bloating, increased constipation or diarrhea and even increases in hunger.

Hydration for Constipation

Consuming water with electrolytes can help rehydrate the body and allow the colon to absorb water more efficiently. It is important to include electrolytes in your water whether you struggle with constipation or diarrhea; the electrolytes will help move nutrients into your cells and help your body adequately absorb the water. The typical recommendation we provide our clients is 80 to 100 ounces (2.4 to 3 L) of water per day, but of course, this depends on several factors, including activity level, caffeine consumption, body size and so on.

If you drink a lot of water and are frequently peeing, consider adding electrolytes to help you absorb the water you are drinking. The water could be going straight through you, which is why you remain thirsty despite efforts to hydrate! The primary electrolytes that your body uses are sodium, potassium, magnesium, calcium, phosphorus, chloride and bicarbonate. (See the Electrolyte Sources section below for electrolyte sources.)

Most of our clients, after focusing on hydration, experience immediate improvements in energy, digestion and overall bloating.

Hydration for Diarrhea

If you experience loose stools or diarrhea, it is also important for you to remain hydrated. You may even need electrolytes more than someone who is experiencing constipation. If you're having diarrhea, especially multiple times a day, the first place to start improving your symptoms is to be sure you are rehydrating yourself.

Electrolyte Sources

You don't have to buy a fancy electrolyte replacement to get the electrolytes you need daily, unless that is your preference. One way to focus on getting enough minerals and electrolytes in your day-to-day life is through the variety of electrolyte-dense foods that you consume.

Foods with electrolytes include:

- Spinach
- Coconut water
- Kale
- Avocados
- Broccoli

- Potatoes
- Beans
- Almonds
- Peanuts
- Soybeans
- Tofu
- Strawberries
- Watermelon
- Fruit juice
- Oranges
- Bananas
- Tomatoes
- Milk
- Yogurt
- Fish
- Turkey
- Chicken
- Veal
- Raisins
- Olives

If you are still experiencing pebbly stool even after focusing on consuming electrolyte-rich foods, consider using an electrolyte addition in your water.

Trace Minerals

Trace minerals can also be important for hydration and digestive function. Trace minerals, also known as microminerals, are inorganic substances that are required by the body to facilitate physiologic functions (including digestion!). We only need "trace" amounts of them daily, but they are vital to overall health and can greatly improve digestion when they are consumed. Trace minerals help with enzyme makeup and some trace minerals are even constituents of hormones.

A few common trace minerals include:

- Iron
- Iodine
- Zinc
- Copper
- Chromium
- Manganese
- Selenium
- Molybdenum

Some common symptoms of trace mineral deficiencies can include:

- Constipation
- Bloating or abdominal pain
- Loss of appetite
- Nausea and vomiting
- Increased muscle cramping

You can find trace minerals as a supplement that you add to water, or there are several herbs rich in minerals that are great to consume as a tea on a regular basis. The herbs that are rich in minerals include:

- Alfalfa
- Dandelion leaf
- Nettles
- Red raspberry leaf

These herbs can be purchased as a loose-leaf herb and made into a tea. When I am purchasing bulk herbs, I like to use Mountain Rose Herbs (mountainroseherbs.com).

The Nervous System and Gut Health

Your nervous system is fundamental when we are thinking about how to improve gut health. When your nervous system is on high alert, your gut is on high alert as well. We talked about the gut–brain connection earlier, but to elaborate on how the brain and our thought patterns specifically influence digestion, we want to hone in on neuroplasticity.

Neuroplasticity describes the ability of the brain to adapt and change. Lifestyle changes and brain exercises can help improve neural connections in your brain to allow it to continue to develop and change. In Appendix C (page 154), you will find an example of a neuroplasticity journal. The journal exercise is designed to rewire and change the way your brain interprets your symptoms.

The research is still very new, but some studies have shown that neuroplasticity and limbic system retraining is helpful for the following things:

- Pain reduction
- Anxiety management
- Stress response
- Mindfulness
- Sleep
- Increased energy

It is amazing that our brains can change and improve neural pathways, but what does this have to do with digestive issues and food sensitivities? The nervous system could be overly sensitive and responsive to certain triggers, even if those triggers aren't a problem anymore. In regard to food and supplements, your nervous system may have learned to associate food, supplements or symptoms like constipation, bloating, gas, and so on with danger. Even if you have taken all the necessary steps to improve your digestive symptoms, the nervous system could still be in charge, leading you to respond to food or symptoms in the way that it has been programmed to in the past.

One of the most powerful things you can do on your digestive health journey is to practice changing the way you think. The overall goal is to rewire the neural pathways and reprogram your responses that have in the past kept you "stuck," even after your body has healed. The neurons that fire together, wire together, which means that we need to focus on rewiring associations that come up when we are thinking about our digestive issues.

If you are inspired to focus on neuroplasticity to improve your digestive health there are some specific action steps you can take. We'll discuss improving your gut-brain connection, lifestyle modifications and dietary additions in the next sections.

Improve Your Gut-Brain Connection

The link between the gut and the brain is powerful, and optimizing the mind *and* the brain is important on any digestive health journey. Because there is constant communication between the gut and the brain, you cannot ignore your thoughts, stress or cognition.

Gratitude

Your mind wants to be negative to protect you from disappointment, but focusing on gratitude is a proven method of reducing stress, overcoming trauma and creating new neural pathways.

Breathwork

Breathwork is one of the quickest ways to take your body from "fight or flight" to "rest and digest." One of my favorite breathwork exercises is called box breathing. It's simple: you breathe in for 4 seconds, hold for 4 seconds, breathe out for 4 seconds and hold for 4 seconds.

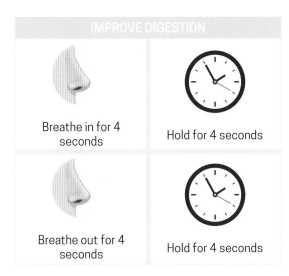

Meditation

As mentioned above, you are programmed to be negative and it takes a lot of work to rewire this thought process. If you sit with your thoughts about your symptoms and see them more like waves in the ocean, coming in to shore and then going back to the ocean, you can acknowledge the thought you are having without taking every thought as the truth. If your nervous system is amped, like a tea kettle about to boil over, you might feel more anxiety at the beginning of the process of trying to improve neuroplasticity. The beginning can be overwhelming if you are not used to sitting quietly and observing your thoughts. Instead of trying to sit down and meditate for 30 minutes when you are just getting started, try 2 minutes at a time to allow the steam to slowly release, instead of boiling over. Meditation is a powerful tool to allow yourself to become an observer of your thoughts. If we are not quiet enough, we remain disconnected from our thoughts and our bodies.

Reframing Your Thoughts

Your thoughts become your feelings and your feelings influence your behavior. If you fear food due to your digestive symptoms, this stress can trigger your nervous system into a fight-or-flight state, leading to the bloat you were trying to avoid. If your wired reaction to sitting down for a meal includes thinking about how bloated you will become, try this instead: "I'm improving my digestive health every day and I know that one day this food will not make me bloated" or "In the past this food has triggered bloat, but that doesn't mean that it will today." If you start with observing your thoughts to just merely see what comes up, you can approach these thoughts without judgment and practice reframing them.

Implement Lifestyle Modifications

Simple daily practices like movement and improving sleep can boost your neuroplasticity without overwhelming you.

Movement

Movement and physical activity have been shown to improve neuroplasticity because they alter the structure and function of synapses in the brain and also increase the density of neurons that impact mood and attention. Movement doesn't have to be intense or stressful and, in fact, focusing on movement that you actually enjoy will allow you to remain consistent. If possible, get outside in the sun for 30 minutes a day and move in a way that is enjoyable to you!

Sleep

Prioritizing sleep and getting 7 to 8 hours of sleep per night is essential for improving the gut–brain connection and neuroplasticity. While sleeping your brain organizes information, "rests and digests" and reduces inflammation. Lack of sleep can contribute to overall inflammation, increased stress hormone production and decreased cognition.

Instead of thinking about what you can take out of your diet, focus on what you can *add* to improve your gut health and improve your symptoms. Some great dietary additions include polyphenols, omega-3 fatty acids and resistant starch. Add these to your diet to encourage the flourishing of your "good" gut bacteria.

Polyphenols

Polyphenols are aromatic compounds found in foods such as fruits, vegetables, whole grains, cocoa, coffee, olives, olive oil and even beverages like black and green tea. These compounds protect plants from ultraviolet radiation and against other pathogens. Polyphenols have been studied and shown to play a protective role in the prevention of cancer, cardiovascular disease, diabetes, osteoporosis and neurodegenerative diseases. In addition, polyphenols reduce inflammation in the body and encourage the growth of "good" bacteria in the gut (like *Bifidobacterium* and *Lactobacillus*). Polyphenols also inhibit the growth of pathogens in the gut, manage blood sugar and help to slow aging. For a complete list of polyphenol -rich foods, see Appendix D (on page 155).

Omega-3 Fatty Acids

Omega-3 fatty acids like those found in salmon are anti-inflammatory to the gut and the brain and some research even shows that omega-3 fatty acids help increase microbial diversity. Consuming omega-3 fatty acids from food is preferred, but if you do not consume fish like salmon two to three times per week, a supplement could be helpful. For a complete list of foods rich in omega-3 fatty acids, see Appendix D (on page 156).

Resistant Starch

Resistant starch is starch molecules that resist digestion and function like a soluble fiber. It is created when starchy foods such as potatoes and rice are cooked and then cooled to room temperature. Resistant starch, although not a prebiotic fiber, acts like a prebiotic and is typically more tolerable than prebiotic fiber for those that are sensitive. One of the main reasons that resistant starch improves so many aspects of health is because it feeds from the good bacteria in the intestine and increases the production of short chain fatty acids like butyrate, which is essential for reducing inflammation in the gut and improving dysbiosis. Including resistant starch can be a great way to start to nourish the good bacteria in the gut while it is still sensitive to prebiotics and working on increasing variety. Resistant starch has been shown to selectively fuel the growth of healthy bacteria in the gut, assist with appetite regulation and improve insulin sensitivity. Resistant starch gives a great excuse for meal prepping in advance. When you cook a sheet pan of potatoes or a pot of rice then let them cool, they develop resistant starch that remains even if you reheat.

For a more comprehensive list, see Appendix D (on page 155).

What You're Eating

Traditionally, the narrative around what to eat for gut health includes a massively long list of restrictions, but I am here to change that narrative. Gut health is about variety and inclusion, not exclusion and restriction. Although there are certain foods that might trigger your symptoms, when your gut is cared for properly, these trigger foods decrease over time, allowing for more variety in your diet and therefore improvement in the composition of your gut bacteria.

Restriction can be a vicious cycle of feeling better, followed by symptoms. Most clients that we work with have been on the merry-go-round of symptoms that has included restricting a food group, finding relief for a few weeks, restricting another food group, finding relief for a few weeks, and so on. By the time they work with us, they are eating a narrow list of foods, still bloated and fearful about whether they will ever feel better.

One question I would encourage you to ask yourself is, "If I am still bloated eating the same five foods, what makes me think that restricting more is going to relieve my symptoms?"

Oftentimes this question brings a huge lightbulb moment. Maybe food restriction is not the answer and there are many other missing pieces to your digestive health puzzle. Food elimination has its time and place, but oftentimes, without the proper foundational support (everything we have discussed up to this point), relief isn't found.

My hope for you as you read this chapter is that you feel encouraged and inspired to add new foods back into your diet, challenge your mindset around why you think you cannot tolerate certain foods, and focus on reintroducing foods slowly to help fuel your gut.

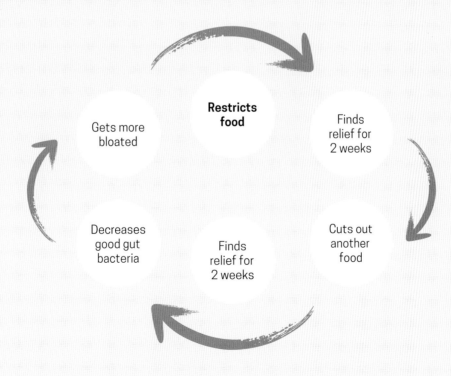

Restricts food → Finds relief for 2 weeks → Cuts out another food → Finds relief for 2 weeks → Decreases good gut bacteria → Gets more bloated

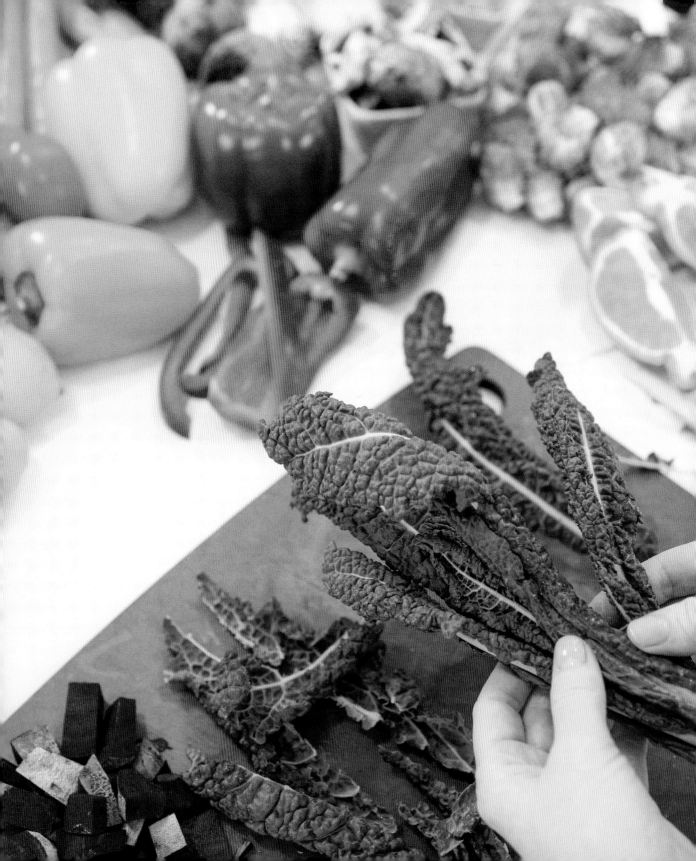

If you learn anything from this chapter, what I want you to take away is that the key to a healthy and happy gut long term (and a wide variety of gut bacteria) is variety on your plate. How does it feel to approach your digestive health from a place of abundance versus restriction? Maybe it makes you excited . . . or maybe it makes you anxious. Either way, hang with me.

What Matters for Gut Health?

Knowing what to eat to improve your gut health can be confusing and probably at times overwhelming. This section is going to highlight a few key components that should always be a consideration in your meals. Focusing on what you can eat and what you can include is the ultimate gut glow-up.

Fiber

What Is Fiber?

You probably know what a big role fiber plays in digestion, but the information out there about fiber can be confusing and controversial. When you hear the word *fiber,* you may also have a visual in your mind of your grandma stirring a thick powder into her orange juice. But fiber isn't just a nasty powder you can mix into a beverage. It is delicious, filling and found in so many different foods. Fiber has three main roles: gut motility, stool consistency and feeding the gut bacteria. We need quite a bit of fiber each day and research shows that Americans only get about half of their recommended daily consumption of fiber. Our fiber goal is 25 to 38 grams a day. Fiber is found in foods like whole grains, vegetables, fruits, legumes, nuts and seeds. Each of these foods contain two types of fiber, both of which play a role in digestive health.

Soluble fiber dissolves in water, forms a gel and helps stool to be soft and well formed. This type of fiber simultaneously helps soften the stool for those who are constipated and also decreases diarrhea. This is also the type of fiber that specifically feeds your gut bacteria.

Some common foods that contain soluble fiber:

- Oats
- Legumes
- Oranges
- Psyllium husk
- Chia seeds
- Flaxseeds
- Avocado

Insoluble fiber does the opposite of soluble fiber and does not dissolve in water and does not create a gel. This type of fiber helps to move things through the colon and acts like a broom.

Some common foods that contain insoluble fiber:

- Skins of fruit and vegetables
- Nuts and seeds
- Beans
- Whole grains
- Wheat bran

Fermentable/Prebiotic Fiber

This type of fiber has been shown to alter gut microbiota by specifically feeding the gut bacteria. As a result, fermentable fiber alters the quantity and variety of good gut bacteria in the gut microbiota. These types of fibers are the food that our gut bacteria feed on, which make them a crucial part of maintaining overall gut health.

Prebiotic Fiber

You may already be frustrated with fiber and associate fiber with an increase in your digestive symptoms. It is common that I hear clients say "The 'healthier' I eat, the worse I feel." Typically, this is because of increased fermentation in the gut (due to fiber) and therefore an increase in bloat. You may also be frustrated by fiber because it has seemed to be the only solution that has been provided to you thus far. "Eat more fiber" or "just take MiraLAX" are common solutions given for digestive problems and when fiber is given as the answer to a slew of digestive problems without any further inquiry, it can actually exacerbate symptoms.

Prebiotics not only feed your gut bacteria, they also are critical to the production of short chain fatty acids. Short chain fatty acids are a byproduct of fermentation in the gut. When your probiotic bugs eat prebiotic fiber, they pay you back by producing short chain fatty acids (like butyrate), which are anti-inflammatory to the gut, the brain and overall to the body. Not only are short chain fatty acids essential for gut health, they are critical for brain health. Short chain fatty acids (also known as postbiotics) are the best kept secret when it comes to gut health and further promote the concept of variety and inclusion versus restriction. The more prebiotic fiber, the more bacterial diversity and the more short chain fatty acid production. A win–win for the gut and the brain.

Some common foods that contain prebiotic fiber:

- Asparagus
- Banana
- Dandelion greens
- Eggplant
- Endive
- Garlic
- Honey
- Jerusalem artichoke
- Jicama
- Kefir
- Leeks
- Legumes
- Onions
- Peas
- Radicchio
- Whole grains
- Yogurt

Now let's talk about *why* fiber can make things worse:

1. If you are already constipated, you want to try to get your bowels moving before you load yourself up with fiber. If your constipation is due to dehydration, the more fiber you eat, the more water is required. So, loading up with fiber without compensating with water can make the constipation problem even worse.

2. Fiber can cause problems if it is added too quickly. Your gut is a muscle and just like every other muscle in the body, needs to be trained slowly. Just as you wouldn't hit your heaviest deadlift after 6 months off at the gym, you don't want to go from 0 to 30 grams of fiber in a day because your system will have a hard time processing and accommodating the fiber.

3. Different types of fiber do different things. If you are avoiding all prebiotic and fermentable fibers because you are worried about symptoms, you could actually be decreasing the overall diversity of bacteria in your gut, which down the road will make your symptoms worse. (Pro Tip: all prebiotics are fiber, but not all fiber is prebiotic.) The live bacteria that you have in your gut need food to survive. And these live bacteria do help with gut motility and the gut–brain connection, so the solution is not to avoid all prebiotic fiber to avoid all bloat. The solution is to add this type of fiber slowly. Remember, even adding 1 tablespoon at a time will be powerful.

4. Some higher-fiber foods contain FODMAPs, which are highly fermentable carbohydrates that can worsen symptoms in those who experience constipation and diarrhea. The small intestine absorbs FODMAPs very poorly, so for those who struggle with small intestinal bacterial overgrowth, FODMAPs can trigger symptoms. This doesn't mean you need to avoid FODMAPs; instead, just be aware that they can increase symptoms, so add them slowly.

5. Just because you cannot tolerate high-fiber foods doesn't mean you should completely avoid them. Elimination can be used to get out of a symptom flare, but avoiding them will restrict growth of beneficial gut bacteria. Being able to liberalize your diet has big-picture benefits for digestive health.

30 Plants per Week

The largest study that has been done on gut health to date has shown that individuals who focus on consuming 30 plants per week in the form of fruits, vegetables, whole grains, nuts, seeds, herbs and spices have overall better gut health. This is an important lightbulb moment and mindset shift for so many individuals struggling with digestive concerns. In thinking about improving gut health, it's important to think about what to include versus what to cut out. Approaching your symptoms and diet from a mindset of inclusion might feel foreign to you, but I promise, your gut bacteria will thank you!

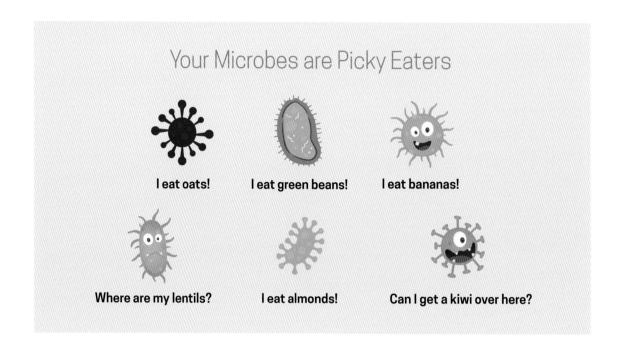

Your Microbes are Picky Eaters

I eat oats!

I eat green beans!

I eat bananas!

Where are my lentils?

I eat almonds!

Can I get a kiwi over here?

Diversity Is the Name of the Game

As humans, we don't naturally produce the enzymes to process fiber—that is what our gut bacteria are there to do. Fiber goes largely undigested until it reaches the large intestine, where your gut bacteria digest this fiber for you. The wider variety of foods you eat, the wider variety of probiotic bacteria that you'll have in your gut and the more benefit you will receive.

Fiber is found in a lot of foods and supplements and the more you can include, the merrier. Although you may initially have symptoms from consuming these foods, you can allow your gut to adapt to digesting them by introducing small amounts (even if just 1 tablespoon) at a time. The overall goal is two to three sources of prebiotic fiber each day. See the list on page 44 for ideas.

Did you know that different fibers from foods feed different bacteria? Simply put, the gut bacteria that prefer asparagus are different from those that prefer bananas. It's good to include as much variety as you can, even if progress is slow. The benefits of variety over time outweigh the in-the-moment comfort of restricting yourself to limited foods that may not cause symptoms but only feed a limited variety of gut bacteria.

Bacterial diversity in your gut is important for:

- Oral tolerance of food
- Immune health
- Optimal hormone function
- Neurological function

If you have low bacterial diversity, you might feel all carbohydrates make you bloated or you have an intolerance to all legumes, beans and so on. Again, temporary relief might be super-satisfying, but over time may be detrimental to overall functioning of the rest of your body.

If you are one to eat the same things all the time out of convenience or preference, don't let this alarm you. There are simple ways to add variety, while still enjoying the foods you love the most. Variety to start could even look like buying one to two different things each week to introduce different sources of fiber into your diet.

Helpful Ways to Add Fiber

Add chia seeds/flaxseeds/hemp seeds/ pumpkin seeds to:

- Scrambled eggs
- Salad dressing
- Nut butter
- Smoothies
- Oatmeal
- Chia pudding
- Yogurt
- Water
- Juice
- Stir-fry
- Salads
- Breads
- Cakes
- Breakfast bars
- Pancakes
- Dips
- Ground meat

Add greens to:

- Egg scrambles
- Smoothies
- Muffins
- Soups
- Casseroles
- Pasta sauce
- Kale chips
- Soups
- Sauces
- Pesto

Prepare root veggies (like sweet potato, parsnips, carrots, beets) different ways:

- Made into fries
- Boiled
- Mashed
- Added to an omelet
- Cooked in a stir-fry
- Made into chips
- Grilled
- Add as a snack with hummus or dip

Consume whole grains (like quinoa, oats, brown rice) these ways:

- Overnight oats
- Brown rice pasta
- Popcorn as a snack
- Grain bowls
- Oats in a smoothie
- Oatmeal energy bites
- Quinoa or oatmeal cookies
- Soups and stews
- Whole grain crackers
- Granola with quinoa and oats

Add legumes (like beans, lentils and peanuts) to:

- Salads
- Bean dips
- Hummus
- Eggs
- Soups
- Stir-fries
- Bean burgers

Prepare cruciferous veggies (cauliflower, Brussels sprouts, broccoli) these ways:

- Steamed and frozen into smoothies
- Puréed into mashed potatoes
- Air fried
- Added to a stir-fry
- Steamed and added to a hummus
- Riced and added to smoothies
- Added to soup
- Mashed and fried into fritters

Use nuts (like almonds, walnuts, pecans and cashews) for:

- Nut butter
- Smoothies
- Salad toppings
- Nut butter sauce (e.g., peanut sauce)
- Grain bowl toppings
- Granola
- Yogurt toppings
- Cereal additions

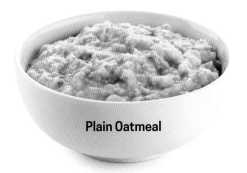

Plain Oatmeal

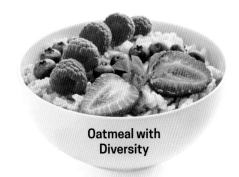

Oatmeal with Diversity

To continue thinking about inclusion versus exclusion, let's use oatmeal as an example. My husband, maybe similar to you, enjoyed his maple and brown sugar oatmeal every morning for about 20 years. Instead of thinking that you must come up with an entirely new breakfast, how can you increase variety while still enjoying your morning bowl of oats? Think about what you can add to your oatmeal to boost the plant points. What about adding some chia seeds, flaxseeds and hemp seeds? Can you slice some fruit and add it to the top? What about some chopped nuts and coconut flakes on top as well? By the time you are finished crafting your perfect bowl of oatmeal, you not only have a work of art, you might also have ten to twelve different plants in just one bowl. Now 30 plants per week doesn't seem so overwhelming, does it? This mindset allows you to still consume your basic favorites, with the added twist of variety.

Decreasing Digestive Distress

Keep in mind that as you introduce new foods into your diet, you may experience some discomfort, especially if you have restricted them for a long time. There are ways in which you can cook and prepare your foods to make them easier to digest:

- Think about including well-cooked vegetables instead of large raw salads

- Consider blending foods like fruit into a smoothie versus eating a whole raw fruit

- Consider adding sprouted forms of whole grains like sprouted oats, wheat and so on to allow for easier digestion (see Appendix E [page 157] for more information)

- Consider adding creamy nut butters and seed butters before whole nuts

- Use sprouting and soaking for legumes and nuts to enhance digestion (see Appendix E on page 157 for a guide on how to do this)

Fermented and Probiotic-Rich Foods

Fermented and probiotic-rich foods have become quite popular, and for good reason. Aside from flavor, there are a lot of reasons to consume probiotic-rich and fermented foods. It is also important to address misconceptions that they are one and the same.

Probiotics

By definition, probiotics are live bacteria (microbes) and must yield some health benefit. For a food to be labeled "probiotic" it must deliver a level of live microbes. The health benefit must be a result in part at least from the presence of microbes. Probiotics are typically found in supplement form and can be taken orally as a capsule or in a powder.

Fermented Foods

Fermented foods are made by live microbes, but live microbes might not survive in the food that you consume post-fermentation. Examples include sourdough, kombucha and so on. Beer and wine undergo a fermentation process but don't have any probiotic activity. In addition, these foods may not have been tested for health benefits beyond basic nutritional value and likely don't meet the bar to actually be a health product. Fermented foods do contribute a diverse array of microorganisms and have the potential to affect health, but we cannot measure the number of bacteria (microbes) that they contain.

Fermented + Probiotic Food

A fermented and probiotic-rich food by definition also must yield some kind of health benefit and the health benefit also must result in part at least from the presence of live microbes. There are several common foods that are fermented and probiotic rich (like yogurt, kefir and certain cheeses). Yogurt meets the qualifications of a fermented probiotic-rich food because it contains acidophilus and acidophilus has been studied for its ability to alleviate constipation and diarrhea.

Why Eat These Foods?

Consuming probiotic and fermented foods in your diet is a great way to introduce beneficial bacteria to the gut without taking another supplement. The digestive tract is home to more than 500 species of bacteria comprising about 100 trillion bugs altogether. To maintain colonization, probiotics must be taken (or eaten) regularly and fed with prebiotics regularly. Probiotics act like travelers. They come into the gut, see the sights, eat the food, then leave.

It is also important to make sure that you are matching the strain to the condition. Every probiotic has a distinct function and health benefit, so it is important that when you are planning to take a probiotic, the strain makes sense for the condition you are experiencing. For example, if you had a migraine, you would go to the pharmacy and ask what medication you needed to take, for how long and at what dose.

The general recommendation for probiotics is to consume between 1 and 25 billion colony-forming units (CFUs). For reference, most store-bought yogurts contain approximately 1 billion CFUs per serving. We can get a lot of probiotics from the food we eat and consuming probiotics from food is a great way to continually introduce beneficial strains daily. You may experience some discomfort when adding probiotic-rich foods to your diet so go slow and allow your digestive tract time to adapt. Consider adding these foods to recipes to start (e.g., using a dollop of probiotic-rich yogurt in a smoothie). There are several recipes in this book that utilize probiotic-rich foods as ingredients and are a great place to start if you don't already consume probiotic-rich foods.

Examples of probiotic-containing foods:

- Buttermilk
- Aged cheeses
- Cottage cheese
- Kefir
- Yogurt

To get maximum benefit from fermented foods, choose those that contain active cultures, especially foods that are raw and unpasteurized. Avoid foods that are heat-treated after fermentation to ensure that more of the good bacteria from fermentation are still around to help your gut. Fermented foods are a fun way to add variety and flavor to your diet and there are several recipes in this book that include these flavors.

Examples of fermented foods:

- Fermented meats and vegetables
- Miso, kimchi, kombucha
- Pickled vegetables
- Sauerkraut

We give our gut bugs a home and in exchange they help us digest food, synthesize vitamins, protect the immune system and protect the gut barrier (which helps our bodies filter and appropriately absorb nutrients).

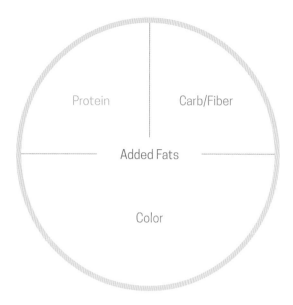

The Gut-Happy Plate: Protein, Fat, Fiber and Color

You have made it all the way through the first parts of this book (or maybe you skipped ahead) and are wondering: What do I eat for gut health? With so much conflicting advice on the Internet, I am here to clear up the confusion.

In general, aim to make your plate look like the plate seen above. Fill half of the plate with colorful fruits and vegetables. Fill one quarter of your plate with protein, and the remaining quarter of your plate with carbs and fiber. Be sure to top everything off with some fat, too!

What if eating for gut health could be more about *inclusion* versus *exclusion*? What if the focus could be on adding enjoyment back into the meals that you miss the most? Eating for your digestive complaints doesn't have to mean eating bland, boring or repetitive food. In fact, it is quite the opposite!

As you have learned from the previous chapters, gut health is about so much more than just what you put on your plate. When the foundational pieces are addressed, your gut can tolerate a lot more variety. So, that being said, if you have skipped to this part of the book, go back and nail the basics first!

Foundationally, I believe that there are a few key pillars for food for gut health:

- Variety
- Diversity of plants
- Blood-sugar balance
- Enjoyment and pleasure

Variety

We have already discussed variety in previous chapters but as you start to make your gut-happy plate, think about what foods you can *add* to your plate versus what you can take away. What toppings, fiber sources, grains, polyphenols, omega-3 fatty acids and resistant starches would complement the meals that you already love?

Diversity of Plants

The gut thrives with diversity. As you start to implement your gut-happy practices, make it a goal to include 30 different plants per week. You can track this using the weekly reflection form in Appendix A (page 151). When you are grocery shopping, try to buy new foods, even if just one or two at a time. One way I have learned to embrace this is by eating seasonally. I love to go to the farmers' market and see what is available at different times of the year. It's fun to get my daughter involved and have her pick out some produce while we shop around.

Blood-Sugar Balance

It's not uncommon that due to restrictive gut-health diets we find blood sugar is very imbalanced. With a small list of foods to eat and little fiber, it is harder to manage blood sugar and the blood-sugar imbalances could be to blame for the symptoms (not the food). Keeping blood sugar balanced is fundamental for gut health because not only does it allow you to fuel yourself adequately and remain satisfied, it also allows you to space your meals out to promote the migrating motor complex.

Carbohydrates are fuel for the cells in your body and your brain and some sugar (from carbs) is needed at all times. Blood sugar is like a wave: it goes up when you eat carbs and it crashes down when insulin helps us move sugar into our cells. We feel our best when we have a rolling blood-sugar wave, just like waves of the ocean coming in and out of shore. Our energy depends on blood-sugar balance and the height and speed of the waves depends on the types of carbohydrates we eat. The depth and speed of the crashes depend on the amount of insulin you produce, which is impacted by your microbiome and your insulin sensitivity. In addition, when blood sugar is imbalanced it impacts insulin and cortisol levels. Cortisol is produced by the adrenal glands due to stress. If you are under a lot of stress, eating three blood sugar–balanced meals a day can help decrease stress and improve your gut symptoms. If blood sugar drops, cortisol spikes and gut symptoms increase. Your stress tolerance will improve when your blood sugar is balanced. Protecting your stress hormones and keeping your thyroid healthy by balancing your blood sugar decreases overall stress on your body and prevents you from having to deal with symptoms like shakiness, nausea, hunger or irritability after or between meals.

When you consume carbohydrates that have fiber, it slows down your blood-sugar response and helps to balance out the blood-sugar waves. When a food is wrapped with fiber, the absorption of sugar is slowed because fiber slows digestion. When you eat to balance your blood sugar, your brain and your body communicate well. You avoid the "2 p.m. slump" and blood sugar–induced mood swings that leave you feeling "hangry." In addition, you can avoid waking up throughout the night by balancing your blood sugar.

You can improve your meal satisfaction by adding protein, fat, fiber and color at your meals. Focus on adding to your meals versus taking away from your meals.

Protein

Protein is the building block of many body tissues and neurotransmitters. It helps to build and maintain lean muscle mass and stimulates metabolism. Protein is important for blood sugar because, just like fat, it doesn't break down into glucose and slows digestion so that you feel satiated longer.

Fat

Fat helps with absorption of fat-soluble vitamins (vitamins A, D, E, K), keeps you satiated and is the building block of hormones. Fat also makes food taste amazing! I have heard fat described as the "magic carpet of food flavoring" and it is true! Adding olive oil, avocadoes or a variety of other fats to your meals greatly enhances the flavor and satisfies your brain in feeling full.

Fibrous Carbs

Your large intestines need fiber and a variety of it. Fiber slows digestion, feeds your gut bacteria and creates a slow and gentle increase in blood sugar. Remember that if you are working on adding fiber because of elimination issues, focus on adding it slowly to decrease symptoms.

Color

Non-starchy vegetables and colorful foods add vitamins, minerals, beauty and texture to your meals. If your fiber source for your meal is colorful already (e.g., you are including a sweet potato or berries) try including a non-starchy green vegetable.

See Appendix F (page 159) for a list of foods that belong in each category.

Enjoyment, Satisfaction and Pleasure

When you eat to balance your blood sugar, your brain and body are satisfied and your hunger and appetite are balanced. Food restriction and lack of enjoyment in your meals can lead to feeling unsatisfied, bingeing and feeling out of control with food. You are a human, not a robot, so expecting yourself to eat "perfectly" all the time or stick to a rigid list of "yes" and "no" foods only backfires later. If you have in the past. Don't allow yourself to label foods as "good" and "bad." Just because a piece of birthday cake does not have fiber, it does not mean you should not eat it. One piece of cake or dessert is not going to derail your blood-sugar balance, especially if you are focused on fueling yourself throughout the day and you eat it without judging yourself. Remember, you can always focus on how you eat regardless of what you are eating. I find this tip especially empowering when out to dinner, traveling or in a place where you can't necessarily choose your own meals. Nutrition is about so much more than just *what* is on your plate. Nutrition is pleasure, enjoyment, memories and experiences. All these things positively impact your gut as well. It's important that you still enjoy the foods you love and participate in nourishing and fun experiences on your gut health journey. Food guilt and stress will do more harm to your gut than the food itself.

Foods to Improve Digestion and Ease Symptoms

Bitter Foods

Bitter foods have been used for years to improve digestion and ease symptoms. The standard American diet is rich with sweet and salty foods, and bitter foods are often the forgotten taste. Bitters can be found in tinctures, but there are whole food sources of bitters that are easy to add to your meals and recipes. Bitter foods improve digestion by stimulating saliva production, which then stimulates the entire digestive process. In addition, bitter foods also help your body stay actively in the parasympathetic "rest and digest" state. Bitters gently "tone" the digestive tract and engage our digestion to do more of the work it was designed to do. As an added benefit, bitters also help to stabilize blood sugar and can help with hunger and appetite. You'll notice that a lot of the recipes in this book contain bitter herbs and foods.

Common bitter foods/herbs include:

- Arugula
- Coffee
- Dill
- Dandelion greens
- Jerusalem artichokes
- Saffron
- Kale
- Sesame seeds
- Turmeric
- Ginger
- Citrus
- Peppermint
- Cocoa
- Eggplant
- Green tea
- Brussels sprouts

Sprouted and Soaked Foods

Sprouting and soaking is a great way to increase nutrient density and absorption and promote optimal digestion. Instead of excluding grains, nuts and seeds that you think you cannot tolerate, try soaking and sprouting them to improve digestibility.

You can soak and sprout foods depending on the type. You can sprout legumes, nuts, seeds and sprout seeds (like alfalfa and broccoli). When you sprout a food, you are mimicking the process of germinating a seed into a plant. The process and soaking time differ based on each individual food, so see Appendix E (page 157) for instructions for individual food items.

When you soak a food, you are breaking down phytic acid, a naturally occurring compound in plants that inhibits the absorption of vitamins and minerals like iron, zinc, calcium and B vitamins. Soaking also aids optimal digestion of foods like beans and legumes because it removes some of the oligosaccharides (the compound in beans and legumes that causes gas and bloating).

Sprouting a food increases nutrient density and can enhance vitamins and minerals such as folate, vitamin C, vitamin A and B vitamins.

Herbs for Bloat Relief

Various herbs can be beneficial for bloat relief and are easy to have on hand if you find yourself needing some extra support. Ginger, peppermint and fennel are some of my favorites.

Ginger eases bloating, cramping and gas because it speeds up the movement of food through the GI tract. If you are dealing with an upset stomach, boil some water and add a ½-inch (1.3-cm) slice of fresh ginger (or ¼ to ½ teaspoon of ground ginger). You can also keep ginger tea on hand as a quick and convenient option. You can also try the Happy Digestion Tea on page 123.

Peppermint is anti-spasmodic and great for bloat relief because it helps to dispel gas. When you feel bloated or gassy you can make a hot cup of peppermint tea or you could use some topical peppermint essential oil (diluted with a carrier oil) directly on your stomach with a heating pad.

Fennel is a helpful herb for bloat relief and can be consumed in the form of tea or from the fennel seeds itself. In several cultures it is traditional to chew fennel seeds after eating to help dispel gas. You can also crush 1 to 2 teaspoons of fennel seeds into boiled water to make tea.

The Gut-Happy Kitchen: Everything You Need to Be Prepared

Whether you are cooking for yourself or a family member, having a stocked pantry and fridge makes those "What do I cook?" nights a lot easier. It's important to stock your kitchen and pantry with some easy staples so that you always feel prepared, even in a pinch. The items below are specific items that I personally keep in my kitchen and pantry to help improve my digestive symptoms and that I enjoy cooking with. These are ingredients that not only your gut loves, but your taste buds will appreciate!

Pantry Staples

Legumes and Beans

Legumes and beans are incredibly shelf stable and an easy fiber addition to any meal. Save time by batch-cooking beans at the beginning of the week to create your favorite grain bowl. Batch cooking beans is also a great way to improve resistant starch intake in your diet. A win–win!

- Dried black beans
- Dried lentils
- Canned chickpeas
- Canned white beans

Nuts and Seeds

Nuts and seeds are fiber powerhouses and easy additions to yogurt, oatmeal, salads, smoothies and granola. Nuts and seeds are also nutritional power-houses that are packed with fat, fiber and protein.

- Chia seeds
- Flaxseeds
- Hemp seeds
- Nut butter
- Walnuts
- Cashews
- Pistachios
- Almonds

Grains

When you are in a hurry, grains are easy to prepare and can add convenience, fiber and versatility to a meal. Grains are another easy meal prep option to make at the beginning of the week for your grain bowls. Again, prepping them ahead is another resistant starch win!

- Sprouted quinoa
- Sprouted oats
- Sprouted rice

Frozen Fruits and Vegetables

For convenience, frozen fruits and vegetables are easy to have on hand for nights when you do not have time to go to the store, or when you need an easy smoothie. The best part is that frozen fruits and vegetables have the same amount of nutrients as fresh and are often cheaper.

Fermented Foods

Fermented foods are versatile and offer so many health benefits. I try to keep at least one of the following on hand at all times:

- Sauerkraut
- Kimchi
- Pickles
- Pickled vegetables

Frozen Fish, Poultry and Meats

Having a freezer with poultry, fish or meat provides for a quick crockpot or instant pot meal when in a bind.

Other Staples

- Eggs
- Apple cider vinegar
- Honey or maple syrup
- Ghee
- Avocado oil
- Olive oil
- Spices and dried herbs
- Coconut aminos
- Mustard
- Nutritional yeast

Your Gut Health Action Plan

Now that you have learned the numerous ways that you can support your gut, it is time to put your knowledge into practice. Spend some time creating your own gut health action plan and use Appendix A (page 151) as a resource.

The key to improving gut health long term is to sustainably and slowly introduce habits that can easily become a part of your lifestyle. Instead of implementing all the action steps at once, build on your plan each week as newly added steps become a habit. Focusing on food is one piece of the puzzle, but implementing the lifestyle modifications is just as important.

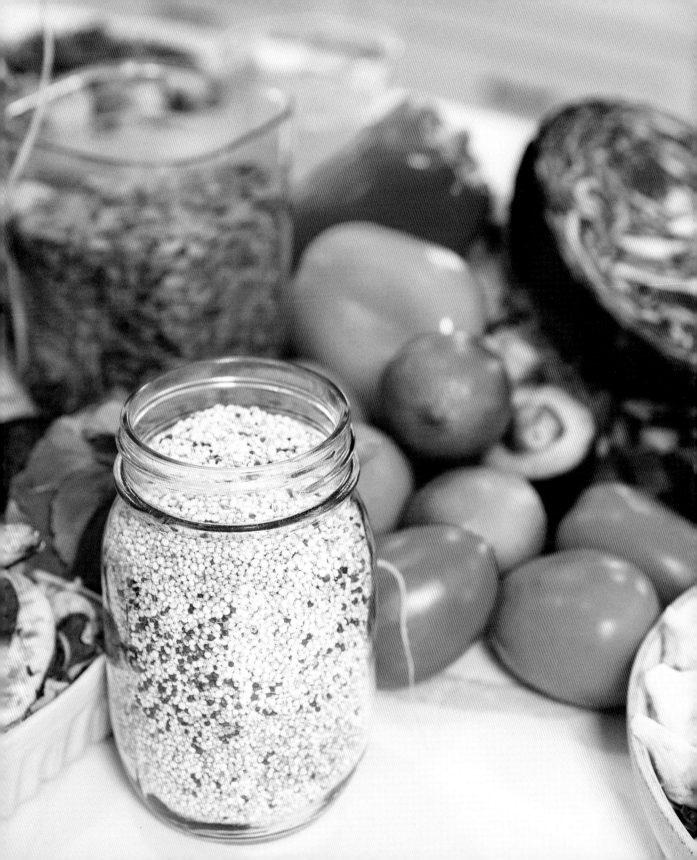

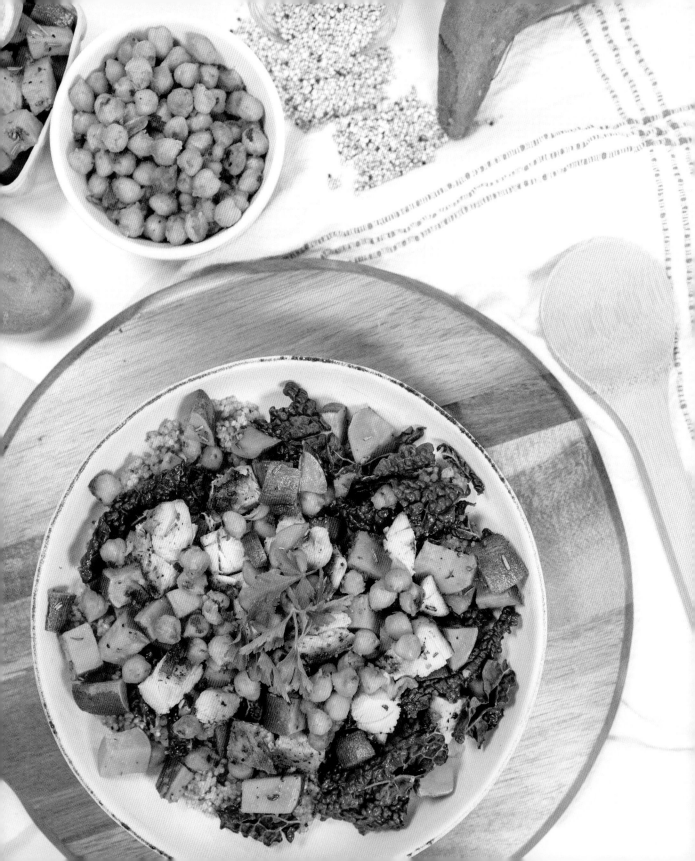

Recipes

I am so excited to share these recipes with you. They are packed with fiber, diversity and flavor. In each recipe you will notice some modifications, substitutions and suggestions. Feel free to utilize these to allow your gut to adapt.

You will also notice that there are some labels. Here is what they all mean:

- **Gluten Free:** Many individuals with digestive issues also have celiac disease or issues with gluten sensitivity. Recipes with this label do not contain gluten and are safe for those with celiac disease.

- **Dairy Free:** Many individuals with digestive issues also have trouble digesting lactose (one of the FODMAPs), which is found in dairy. For many, using lactose-free dairy is an easy swap. If you cannot tolerate any dairy (even lactose free), look for recipes labeled dairy free.

- **High Fiber:** Fiber is a great tool for balancing blood sugar, feeding gut bacteria and keeping you full and satisfied. If you are struggling to digest fiber, please note that you may want to go slow with these recipes and allow your gut to adapt as you increase your fiber intake.

- **Vegan:** Plant-based diversity is a cornerstone for digestive health. Including more plant-based meals can greatly improve digestive health. Recipes with this label are completely plant based with no animal protein.

- **Fermented:** Fermentation is a great way to improve nutrient absorption, improve digestion and include more flavor in your meals. If you are sensitive to fermented foods, please note the fermentation label. If you are working on adding more probiotic-rich and fermented foods, look for recipes with this label.

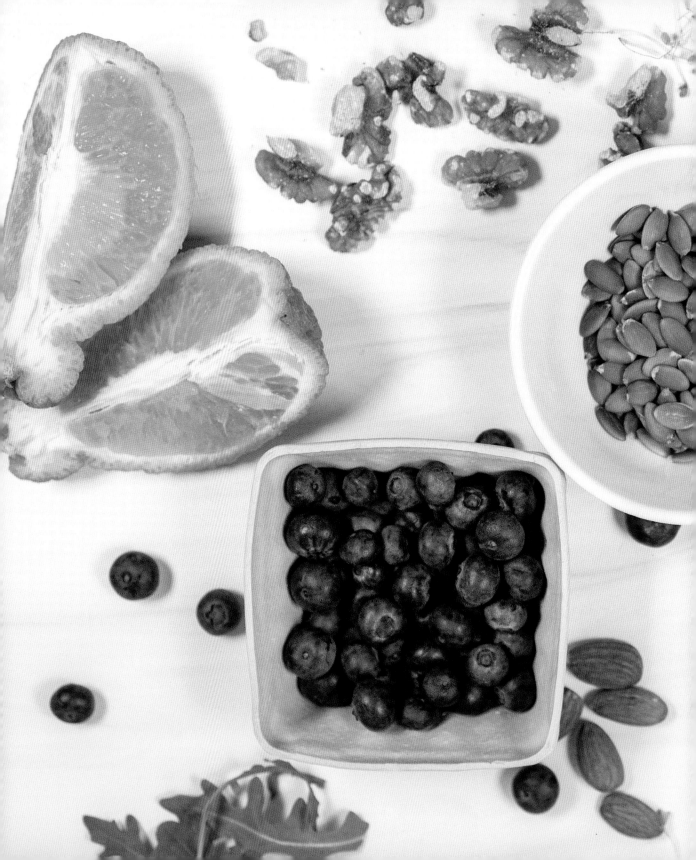

Fiber-Fueled
Breakfasts

Starting your day with fiber and balanced blood sugar is essential for gut health, promoting great sleep, hormone health and feeling energized throughout the day. For many, the mornings are rushed and it's easy to make the excuse of "I didn't have time for breakfast." For that reason, this book contains super-easy recipes that can be prepared the night before or even on the weekend so you can prioritize your breakfast in the morning, regardless of how busy you are.

If you have ever experienced that 2 p.m. "I need chocolate or coffee now" feeling, often that has to do with what you did (or didn't) have at breakfast. Prioritizing protein, fat, fibrous carbs and color at breakfast can be a great way to bypass the 2 p.m. slump and feel energized all day long.

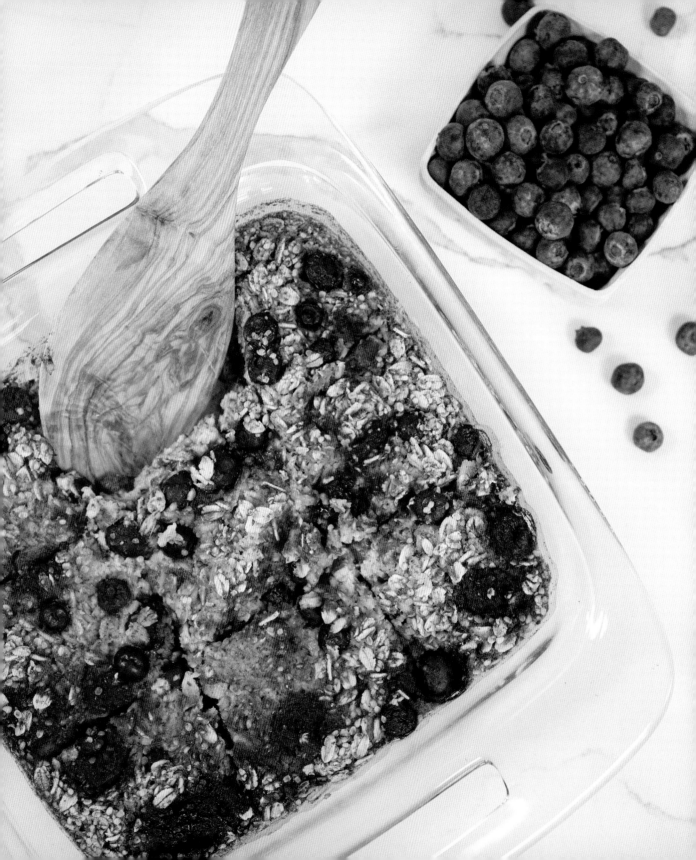

Berry Baked Oatmeal

2 cups (480 ml) almond milk or milk of choice

½ cup (120 ml) unsweetened applesauce

¼ cup (60 ml) maple syrup

2 cups (180 g) rolled or sprouted oats

⅓ cup (45 g) ground flaxseed

⅓ cup (53 g) hemp seeds

1 tsp cinnamon

1½ cups (280 g) frozen mixed berries

This breakfast oatmeal bake is a great meal prep option for breakfast or even for snacks throughout the week. With all the flavorful berries, it's almost like a cobbler for breakfast. It is great topped with Greek yogurt for some extra protein and a probiotic punch.

Oatmeal, applesauce, flax and berries are all prebiotic fibers that feed the "good," beneficial bacteria in the gut, promoting optimal diversity, which has been shown to improve symptoms such as constipation, diarrhea and bloat. Berries also contain a compound called polyphenols, which are packed with antioxidants and can help reduce inflammation in the gut.

Makes 8 servings

Preheat the oven to 350°F (175°C).

In a mixing bowl, combine the milk, applesauce and maple syrup. After the wet ingredients are combined, stir in the oats, flaxseed, hemp seeds and cinnamon. Fold in the frozen berries.

Transfer the mixture to an 8 x 8-inch (20 x 20-cm) baking dish and bake for 40 to 45 minutes, or until the oatmeal is spongy to the touch (and a toothpick inserted into the center comes out clean). Let the baked oatmeal cool slightly. Serve and enjoy warm or store in the fridge for an easy breakfast for up to 5 days.

Notes:

- Use any fruit you enjoy instead of berries.
- Use ground chia seeds instead of flaxseeds.
- If you prefer the oatmeal to be less sweet, use less maple syrup.
- Use sprouted oats for easier digestibility.

Gluten Free, Dairy Free, High Fiber, Vegan

Overnight Oats Four Ways

Overnight oats are a no-cook form of oatmeal that can conveniently be prepped the night before or on the weekend so that when you wake up for a busy day, you have a fiber-filled and delicious breakfast ready to fuel your morning (or even a satisfying snack!). You can eat overnight oats cold, or heat them up—whatever you prefer! Preparing oats this way is an excellent way to include more resistant starch in your daily intake.

Once you prep the base recipe, you can easily create variety in flavor by adding different ingredients. Below you will find four variations of one of my favorite breakfast staples.

Makes 2 servings

Base Ingredients

1 cup (90 g) rolled or sprouted oats

1¼ cups (300 ml) almond milk (or milk of choice)

2 tbsp (22 g) chia seeds

Carrot Cake

½ medium carrot, grated

½ tsp cinnamon

¼ tsp ground ginger

2 tbsp (30 ml) maple syrup

2 tbsp (30 ml) coconut yogurt

2 tbsp (28 g) walnuts, chopped

Chocolate Peanut Butter

2 tbsp (32 g) peanut butter

2 tbsp (14 g) cacao powder

⅓ cup (80 ml) Greek yogurt

2 tbsp (30 ml) maple syrup

Pinch of salt

2 tbsp (20 g) peanuts, chopped (optional)

Cherry Almond

¼ cup (30 g) sliced almonds, toasted

¼ cup (40 g) cherries, diced

⅓ cup (80 ml) plain Greek yogurt

2 tbsp (30 ml) honey or maple syrup

½ tsp vanilla extract

¼ tsp almond extract

Pinch of salt

Savory Chickpea

¼ cup (8 g) chopped spinach or kale

1 tbsp (5 g) nutritional yeast

¼ tsp turmeric

⅓ cup (55 g) canned chickpeas

1 tbsp (15 ml) tahini, plus more for topping (optional)

Pinch of pepper

Pinch of salt

Optional toppings: cilantro, green onions, almonds, cashews

Add the base ingredients (oats, almond milk and chia seeds) to a mason jar or container with a lid. Mix well. Add the ingredients for your desired variation (see below). Cover and place in the fridge overnight or for at least 8 hours.

Remove the oats from the fridge and divide into two jars.

For the Carrot Cake oats:

Add the grated carrot, cinnamon, ground ginger and maple syrup to the base ingredients before putting in the fridge overnight. After removing from the fridge add the yogurt and walnuts.

For the Chocolate Peanut Butter oats:

Add the peanut butter, cacao powder, Greek yogurt, maple syrup and salt to base ingredients before putting in the fridge overnight. After removing from the fridge, top with chopped peanuts, if desired.

For the Cherry Almond oats:

Add the almonds, cherries, yogurt, honey or maple syrup, vanilla and almond extracts and salt to the base ingredients before putting in the fridge overnight.

For the Savory Chickpea oats:

Add the spinach or kale, nutritional yeast, turmeric, chickpeas, tahini, pepper and salt to the base ingredients before putting into the fridge overnight. After removing from the fridge top with optional toppings and extra tahini, if desired.

*See image on page 57.

Notes:

For easier digestibility:

- Use sprouted oats.
- Use lactose-free yogurt if needed (or dairy free yogurt).
- Sauté the spinach or kale for the savory oats first.
- If you are celiac or gluten sensitive, make sure to purchase certified gluten free oats.

Base Ingredient

1 sweet potato

Avocado and Sprouts (for 1 slice)

1 tsp extra virgin olive oil

Pinch of salt

½ avocado, thinly sliced

1 radish, thinly sliced

2 tbsp (7 g) Broccoli Sprouts (see page 145 for recipe)

Juice of ½ a lime

Red pepper flakes, optional

Banana Nut (for 1 slice)

2 tbsp (32 g) nut butter of choice

2 tbsp (20 g) hemp seeds

1 tbsp (11 g) chia seeds

½ banana, sliced

Drizzle of honey

Chia and Coconut (for 1 slice)

2 tbsp (30 g) Chia Jam (see page 139)

1 tbsp (6 g) coconut flakes

Gluten Free, Dairy Free, High Fiber, Vegan

Sweet Pota-Toast Trio

This flavorful take on the ever-popular avocado toast is a crowd favorite, a great way to add color to your morning, and an excellent swap for those who cannot tolerate gluten-containing bread. These toasts are quick to prepare and super flavorful additions to a breakfast.

Makes 3 servings

Trim the ends off the sweet potato. Cut the sweet potato lengthwise into ¼-inch (6-mm) slices to create long toast-like pieces.

Place the sweet potato slices in a toaster and toast twice or until golden brown. You may also set your oven to broil and broil on a baking sheet for 3 to 6 minutes per side or until golden brown.

Allow the sweet potato to cool slightly, then add the toppings you have chosen (see below) and enjoy!

For the Avocado and Sprouts pota-toast:

Drizzle the olive oil on the sweet pota-toast and sprinkle the salt on top of the olive oil. Spread the sliced avocado over the olive oil and salt and top with the radish, Broccoli Sprouts and a squeeze of lime. For extra spice, add a pinch of red pepper flakes.

For the Banana Nut pota-toast:

Generously spread the nut butter over the sweet potato. Add the hemp seeds and chia seeds. Place the sliced banana on the nut butter and seeds and then drizzle with honey to finish.

For the Chia and Coconut pota-toast:

Generously spread the Chia Jam on the toasted sweet potato. Sprinkle with the coconut flakes to finish.

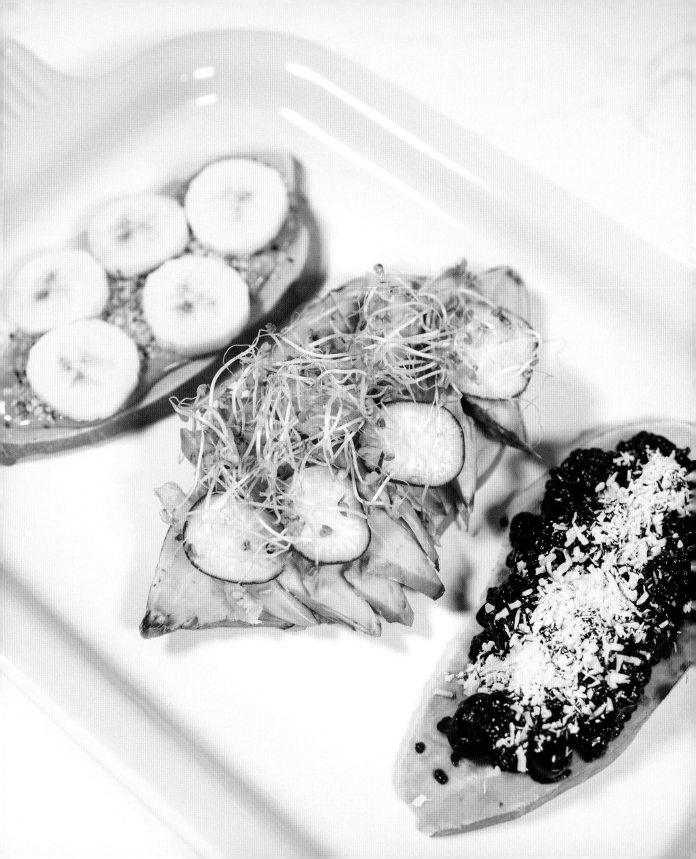

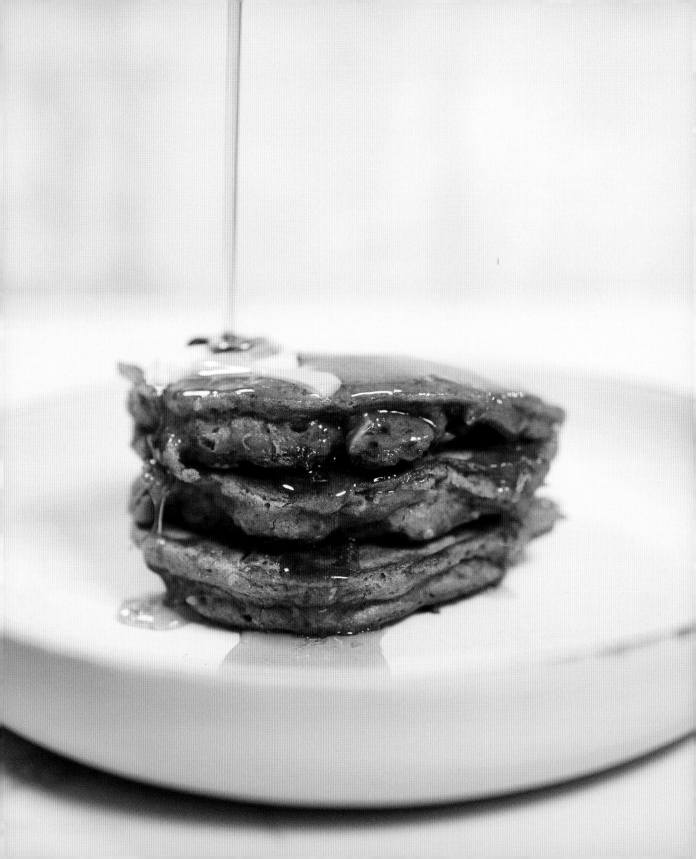

1 tsp baking powder

½ cup (55 g) chopped pecans

1 tbsp (10 g) flaxseeds

1 tsp cinnamon

¼ tsp salt

¾ cup (180 ml) almond milk (or another nut milk)

2 eggs

1 tbsp + 1 tsp (20 ml) coconut oil, melted and divided

1 tbsp (15 ml) apple cider vinegar

¾ cup (184 g) sweet potato purée

Nutty Sweet Potato Pancakes

Sunday mornings aren't complete without a stack of pancakes, at least in my household! These sweet potato pancakes are an amazing twist on the original and perfect for a cool, fall morning. You can roast sweet potatoes to make your own purée or you can use canned for a quick and convenient option. Either way, you are sure to love these super fluffy, nutty pancakes.

Makes 4 servings

In a medium bowl, combine the baking powder, pecans, flaxseeds, cinnamon and salt. In a large bowl, whisk the almond milk, eggs, 1 tablespoon (15 ml) of the coconut oil, apple cider vinegar and sweet potato purée until the eggs and sweet potato purée are combined. Add the dry ingredients to the wet ingredients and whisk until smooth.

In a large skillet over medium-high heat, warm 1 teaspoon of coconut oil. Pour about ¼ cup (60 ml) of the batter onto the oiled pan. Cook the pancake for 2 to 3 minutes (or until the pancake starts to bubble and is solid on one side), then flip and repeat.

Serve and enjoy!

> Note:
>
> Top these pancakes with Chia Jam (page 139)—you won't regret it!

Gluten Free, Dairy Free, Vegan

Base Ingredients

1 cup (240 ml) unsweetened almond milk

¼ cup (44 g) chia seeds

Almond Chocolate

1 tbsp (7 g) cacao powder

1 tbsp (15 ml) maple syrup

¼ tsp vanilla extract

¼ cup (23 g) sliced almonds

Strawberries and Cream

¼ cup (36 g) fresh strawberries

¼ cup (60 ml) full-fat coconut milk (refrigerated overnight)

¼ tsp vanilla extract

⅛ tsp finely grated lemon zest

Banana Crunch

¼ tsp vanilla extract

½ banana, sliced

¼ cup (25 g) Cashew Crunch High Fiber Granola (page 125)

Gluten Free, Dairy Free, High Fiber, Vegan

Chia Pudding Four Ways

Enjoy this delicious, fiber-filled breakfast or snack four different ways! For many of my clients, the key to success on their gut journey is convenience—and chia pudding provides just that. For a quick breakfast or fast and filling snack, this base recipe can easily be adapted to satisfy your taste buds in a variety of ways. No matter the cause of your digestive struggles, chia seeds are your new best friend.

Makes 1 serving

Matcha

¼ cup (60 ml) full-fat coconut milk (refrigerated overnight)

1 tbsp (6 g) matcha powder

¼ avocado

1 tbsp (15 ml) maple syrup

Add the almond milk and chia seeds to a jar with a lid. Stir until the mixture is combined. Add the ingredients for your desired variation (see below). Then place in the fridge to thicken up for at least 4 hours (or overnight for best results).

For the Almond Chocolate chia pudding:

Before adding the base ingredients to the fridge, add the cacao powder, maple syrup and vanilla. Mix well and place in the fridge. Before eating, top with the almonds.

For the Strawberries and Cream chia pudding:

Before adding the base ingredients to the fridge, add the strawberries, coconut milk, vanilla and lemon zest. Mix well and place in the fridge.

For the Banana Crunch chia pudding:

Before adding the base ingredients to the fridge, add the vanilla and banana. Mix well and place in the fridge. Before eating, top with the granola.

For the Matcha chia pudding:

Add the coconut milk, matcha powder, avocado and maple syrup to a blender or food processor. Mix until smooth and combined. Place the matcha mixture into the fridge to thicken for 10 to 15 minutes. Once the mixture has thickened up, add it to the chia pudding base ingredients and refrigerate overnight.

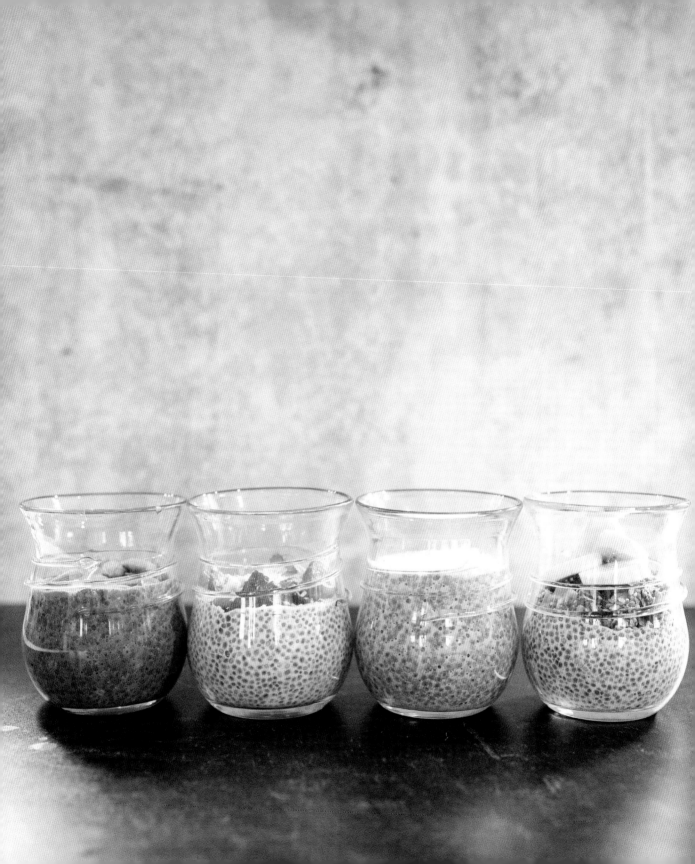

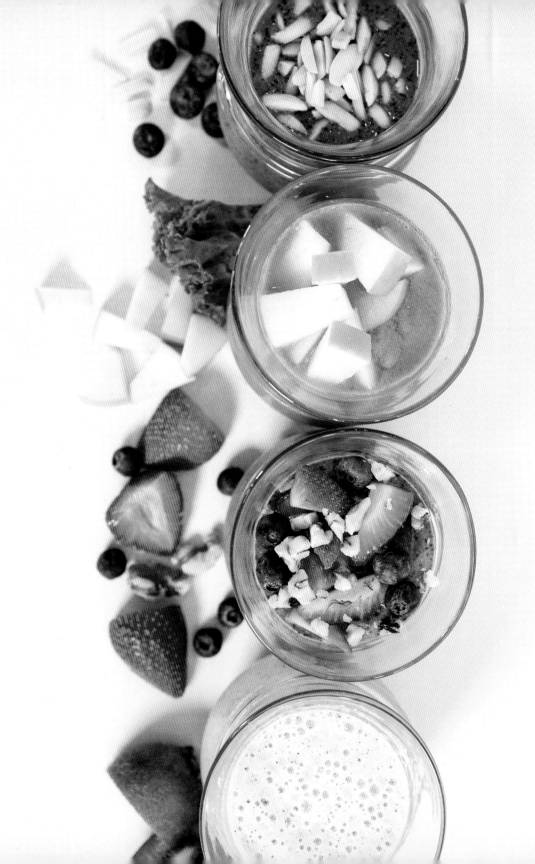

Sips That
Satisfy

Smoothies are a fast, easy and convenient way to pack a lot of nutrition into one cup. Most days, you will find me drinking a smoothie either for breakfast or for a snack. When protein, fat, fiber and color are included, smoothies can be a great way to balance blood sugar, provide tons of nutrition to the gut and give you sustained energy. For many people with digestive issues, smoothies are a great way to try adding in new foods. If you are working on increasing variety in your diet, challenge yourself to put 1 to 2 tablespoons (15 to 30 ml) of something new into your smoothie; your gut will thank you! For a probiotic punch, add 2 tablespoons (30 ml) of kefir to each smoothie or replace half of the suggested milk with kefir.

Anatomy of a Smoothie

I have included several of my favorite smoothie recipes in this book, but don't hesitate to make your own creation. To focus on blood sugar balance and fueling the gut, use this simple outline:

Choose 1 cup (150 g) of fresh/frozen fruit (banana, berries, pineapple, mango, etc.)

Choose 1–2 cups (30–60 g) leafy greens (kale, spinach, chard, etc.)

Choose 1–2 tbsp (10–20 g) seeds (ground flax, chia, hemp, etc.)

Choose 1–2 tbsp (15–30 g) creamy nut/seed butter (almond, coconut, walnut, pumpkin seed, peanut, etc.)

Choose 1 protein (6 oz [15–20g] organic Greek yogurt, collagen peptides, protein powder, tofu, etc.)

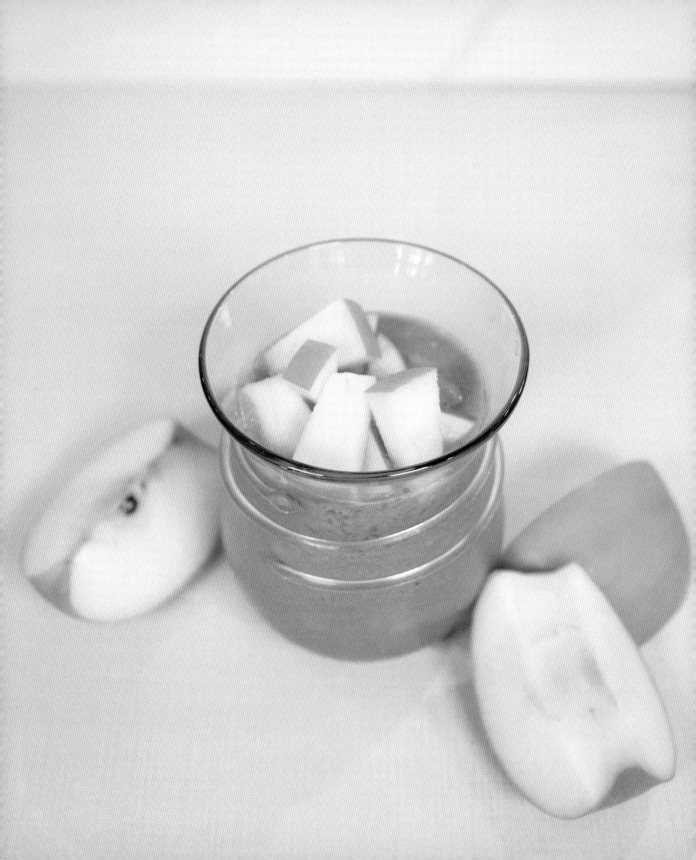

2 bananas, chopped and frozen

4 cups (80 g) kale, frozen or fresh

1 avocado

2 tbsp (20 g) collagen powder (or unflavored protein powder)

1½ cups (360 ml) almond milk (or milk of choice)

2 tbsp (18 g) almonds

2 tbsp (20 g) hemp seeds

2 tbsp (30 ml) Kefir (page 147; optional)

Green Goddess Smoothie

This smoothie packs tons of vitamins and fiber on top of the probiotics from the kefir and the fat your brain loves from the avocado. Enjoy this as a breakfast addition or a midafternoon snack.

Makes 2 servings

Place all the ingredients in a blender and blend until smooth. Pour into a glass and enjoy!

Gluten Free, Dairy Free, High Fiber, Fermented

1½ cup (300 g) frozen berries

1 cup (240 ml) plain Kefir (page, or almond milk; see Note)

½ banana, frozen

2 tbsp (22 g) chia seeds

2 tbsp (20 g) collagen powder (or unflavored protein powder)

Gluten Free, Dairy Free, High Fiber, Fermented

Very Berry Probiotic Smoothie

If you love berries, you will love this probiotic-rich berry smoothie. And spoiler alert, this same recipe can be used to make Probiotic Fruit Pops (see page 129), which are the most refreshing snack on a hot day.

Makes 2 servings

Place all the ingredients in a blender and blend until smooth. Pour into a glass and enjoy!

*See image on page 72.

> Note:
>
> If you cannot tolerate kefir, substitute almond milk or start with 1 to 2 tablespoons (15 to 30 ml) of kefir (and the rest almond milk) and work your way up to tolerating the full amount as your gut allows.

1 cup (155 g) frozen blueberries

1 cup (123 g) frozen cauliflower

½ cup (120 ml) plain Greek yogurt

¼ cup (40 g) vanilla protein powder

2 tbsp (20 g) flaxseeds

1 lemon, juiced

1 cup (240 ml) almond milk

Gluten Free, High Fiber, Fermented

Blueberry Flax Smoothie

This creamy blueberry smoothie is loaded with polyphenols to fuel your gut bacteria. Before the cauliflower scares you off, trust me on this one—the fiber-filled addition adds extra creaminess to the smoothie that you (and your gut!) will love. In addition to the polyphenols in this smoothie you will also have tons of fiber from the flaxseeds and fruits and veggies.

Makes 2 servings

Place all the ingredients in a blender and blend until smooth. Pour into a glass and enjoy!

*See image on page 72.

> Note:
>
> If you do not tolerate large amounts of cauliflower, start with ¼ cup (30 g) or less and slowly increase as your gut allows.

2 kiwis, peeled and sliced

2 tbsp (12 g) rolled or sprouted oats

1 banana, frozen

1 cup (240 ml) almond milk (or milk of choice)

¼ cup (60 ml) Kefir (page 147) or Greek yogurt

1 (¼-inch [6-mm]) piece fresh ginger, grated

Honey, optional, for garnish

Kiwi Ginger Smoothie

Kiwi, oats and ginger are all gut-loving ingredients, especially for getting things moving along. Feel free to adjust the amount of ginger to your preference and add the kefir as you tolerate it.

Makes 2 servings

Place the kiwis, oats, banana, almond milk, kefir or Greek yogurt and ginger in a blender and blend until smooth. Pour into a glass and enjoy! Top with honey if desired.

Note:

If you cannot tolerate kefir, substitute almond milk or start with 1 to 2 tablespoons (15 to 30 ml) of kefir (and the rest almond milk) and work your way up to tolerating the full amount as your gut allows.

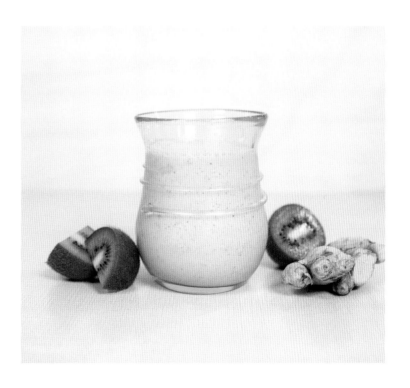

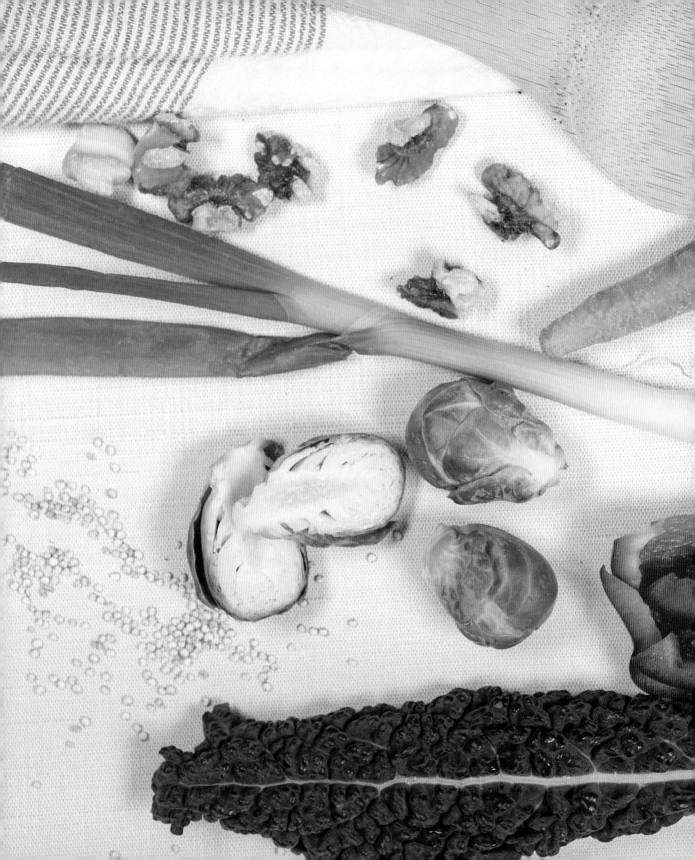

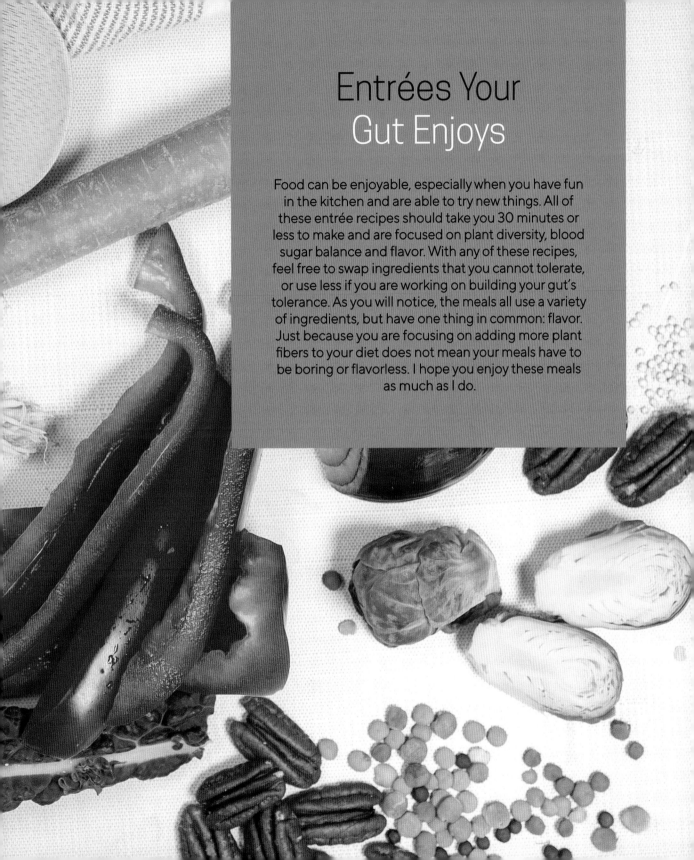

Entrées Your
Gut Enjoys

Food can be enjoyable, especially when you have fun in the kitchen and are able to try new things. All of these entrée recipes should take you 30 minutes or less to make and are focused on plant diversity, blood sugar balance and flavor. With any of these recipes, feel free to swap ingredients that you cannot tolerate, or use less if you are working on building your gut's tolerance. As you will notice, the meals all use a variety of ingredients, but have one thing in common: flavor. Just because you are focusing on adding more plant fibers to your diet does not mean your meals have to be boring or flavorless. I hope you enjoy these meals as much as I do.

Roasted Lemon Chicken

4 chicken thighs, bone-in, skin-on

2 tbsp (30 ml) avocado oil

2 lemons, juiced and zested + 1 lemon, thinly sliced

2 tbsp (11 g) dried oregano

2 tbsp (3 g) dried parsley

½ tsp salt

¼ tsp pepper

1 tbsp (15 g) minced garlic (if tolerated)

This chicken is super fresh, juicy and tender and is the easiest protein addition to any meal. The acidity of the lemon helps to balance the flavor of the chicken and also helps to induce salivation, which improves digestion. For quick and easy grain bowls during the week, prep this chicken ahead, cut it up and have it on hand in the fridge.

Makes 4 servings

Preheat the oven to 350°F (175°C).

Place the chicken thighs, skin-side down, in a baking dish.

Whisk the avocado oil, lemon juice and zest, oregano, parsley, salt, pepper and garlic. Place the lemon slices on top of the chicken. Pour the lemon juice mixture on top of the chicken.

Bake the chicken for 25 minutes or until the chicken is cooked through to 165°F (75°C). Let the chicken rest for 5 minutes, then remove the skin and bones and chop or serve whole.

*See image on page 81.

Note:

Omit the garlic if you do not tolerate it, or use a smaller amount.

Gluten Free, Dairy Free

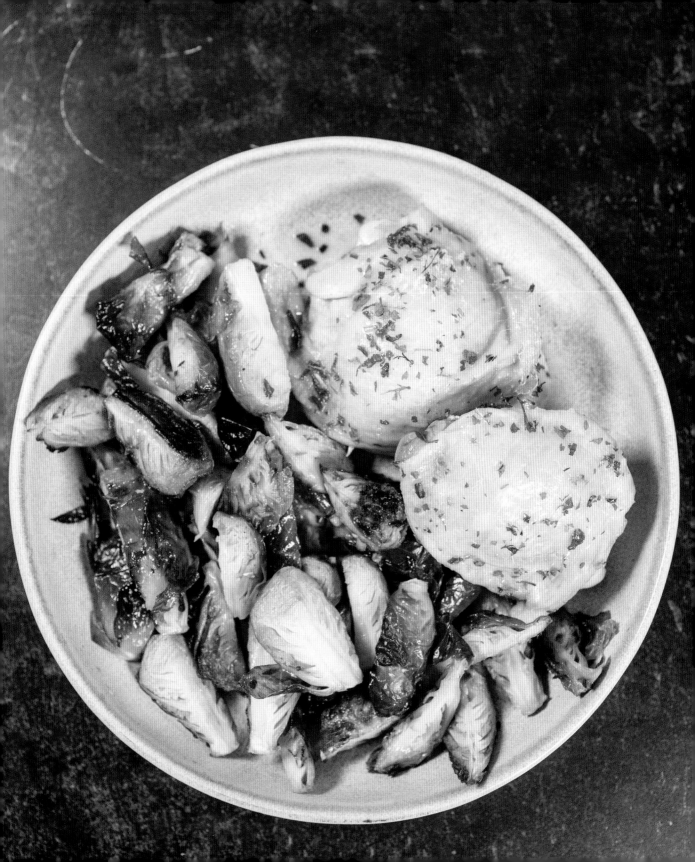

2 lb (907 g) Brussels sprouts

6 tbsp (90 ml) avocado oil (see Note)

½ tsp chili powder (omit if needed)

Himalayan pink salt, to taste

Pepper, to taste

3 limes, zested and juiced

3 tbsp (45 ml) honey

Crispy Honey Lime Brussels Sprouts

There is a restaurant near my house that makes honey lime Brussels sprouts that are my absolute favorite! My mission for this recipe was to re-create my favorite dish—focusing on gut-loving ingredients, of course! If you have an air fryer, I highly recommend crisping the Brussels sprouts in the air fryer; the extra crunch makes them delicious!

Makes 4 servings

Trim and quarter the Brussels sprouts lengthwise and place in a medium mixing bowl.

In another mixing bowl, combine the avocado oil, chili powder, salt, pepper, lime juice and honey. Stir well to combine, then pour about half of the sauce on the Brussels sprouts and mix until all the sprouts are coated well. Set the remaining marinade aside.

To make the Brussels sprouts on the stove, sauté them over medium heat until they are browned and crispy, about 10 minutes.

To make the Brussels sprouts in an air fryer, cook at 400°F (205°C) for 5 to 7 minutes, or until crispy.

After the Brussels sprouts are cooked and crispy, pour the reserved marinade mixture over them and serve with Roasted Lemon Chicken (page 80) on top, or as a side to another favorite dish.

> Note:
>
> If you are cooking this recipe on the stove instead of in an air fryer, you can use olive oil instead of the avocado oil if you would like, as it will be cooking over a lower heat.

Gluten Free, Dairy Free

Marinade

¼ cup (60 ml) avocado oil

½ tsp salt

¼ tsp pepper

½ tsp turmeric

Juice of 1 lemon (approximately ¼ cup [60 ml])

1 tsp dried oregano

Chicken and Sweet Potatoes

2 medium sweet potatoes, cut into ½-inch (1.3-cm) cubes (approximately 4 cups [525 g])

4 boneless chicken thighs

Quinoa

½ cup (85 g) quinoa (see Notes)

1 cup (240 ml) water or Gut-Happy Broth Base (page 119)

¼ tsp salt

Sweet Potato and Chicken "Cha Cha" Bowls

Grain bowls are a staple meal at my house and this is our family's spin on a traditional grain bowl. This bowl is particularly special because it is my daughter's favorite ("Cha Cha" is her nickname!).

What I love the most about grain bowls is that you can easily prepare most of the ingredients ahead and have leftovers for days (switch up the sauce to change the flavor, if desired).

This savory and satisfying bowl is filled with tons of fiber from the quinoa, chickpeas, potatoes and kale, and the plant diversity will help fuel your digestive health and keep your "good" gut bugs happy. If you are working on reintroducing foods into your diet, this recipe offers a lot of flexibility for adding in smaller amounts of ingredients or foods that you may not have previously tolerated.

Makes 6 servings

Preheat the oven to 425°F (220°C).

To make the marinade, in a small bowl, whisk together the avocado oil, salt, pepper, turmeric, lemon juice and oregano.

Spread the sweet potato cubes evenly across a baking sheet. Nestle the chicken thighs between the sweet potatoes and then pour the marinade over the chicken and sweet potatoes. Bake for 35 minutes or until chicken reaches 165°F (75°C) with an instant-read thermometer and the sweet potatoes are tender. Let cool slightly, then chop the chicken and remove the skin if desired.

While the chicken is cooking, prepare the quinoa with the water or Gut-Happy Broth Base and salt according to the package instructions.

(continued)

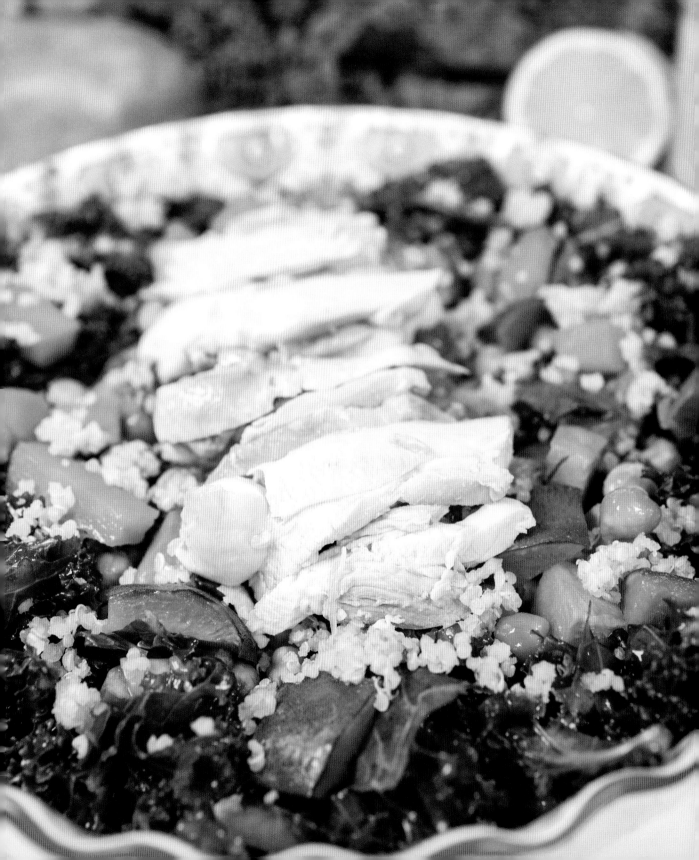

Toasted Chickpeas

1 (15.5-oz [439-g]) can chickpeas (see Notes)

1 tbsp (15 ml) avocado oil

½ tsp salt

¼ tsp pepper

¼ tsp cumin

½ tsp chili powder, optional

Tuscan Kale

1 tbsp (15 ml) avocado oil

4 cups (268 g) chopped Tuscan kale, stems removed (see Notes)

½ tsp salt

Tahini Sauce

¼ cup (60 ml) avocado oil

Juice of 1 lemon (approximately ¼ cup [60 ml])

1 tsp maple syrup

2 tbsp (30 ml) warm water

¼ cup (60 ml) tahini (sesame paste)

Garnish (optional)

1 bunch Italian parsley, chopped

To make the chickpeas, drain, rinse and dry the chickpeas with a paper towel. Add the avocado oil to a medium sauté pan over medium heat and when it is warm, add the chickpeas. Season with the salt, pepper and cumin. For added spice add the chili powder. Sauté until fragrant, approximately 5 minutes, then set aside in a bowl.

In the same pan (with chickpeas removed) prepare the kale. Add the avocado oil over medium heat. When the oil is hot, add the kale and sauté until wilted, 2 to 3 minutes. Sprinkle with the salt. Remove from the heat and set aside in a bowl.

To make the tahini sauce, in a small bowl, whisk the avocado oil, lemon juice, maple syrup, water and tahini until creamy. Add additional tablespoons (15 ml) of hot water one at a time if necessary to allow tahini to mix well.

Assemble the bowls by layering the quinoa, kale, sweet potatoes, chicken and tahini sauce, and finish with a sprinkle of the parsley if desired.

Notes:

Prep ahead: To save time, prep the tahini sauce and quinoa ahead of time. Both will save in the fridge, covered, for up to 5 days.

For easier digestibility:

- Use sprouted quinoa instead of regular quinoa.

- You may also cook the quinoa with the juice of 1 lemon to help with tolerance and breakdown.

- Omit the kale or use a green that you tolerate.

- Use Sprouted Chickpeas (page 143).

2 tbsp (30 ml) avocado oil

1 yellow onion, diced

8 oz (226 g) cremini mushrooms, quartered

2 cloves garlic, minced

½ tsp of salt

¼ tsp pepper

¼ cup (60 ml) apple cider vinegar

1 cup (192 g) green lentils, rinsed

2 cups (480 ml) Gut-Happy Broth Base (page 119) or vegetable broth

8 oz (226 g) egg noodles

1 cup (240 ml) full-fat probiotic yogurt (I used Nancy's organic)

Italian parsley, for garnish

Creamy Lentil and Mushroom Stroganoff

This recipe is a spin on the traditional beef stroganoff. Utilizing high-fiber lentils and mushrooms, your gut is sure to be happy and your taste buds satisfied. In addition to all the plant fiber included, this recipe also uses probiotic-rich yogurt to add creaminess and probiotics to the sauce. This recipe is made with an Instant Pot® but could easily be adapted for the stove by cooking the lentils separately, then adding them to the rest of the sauce ingredients.

Makes 6 servings

Add the avocado oil, onion, mushrooms and garlic to an Instant Pot on sauté mode. Sauté until the onion is translucent and mushrooms are soft, approximately 5 minutes. Sprinkle with the salt and pepper.

Add the apple cider vinegar to the Instant Pot along with the lentils and the Gut-Happy Broth Base or vegetable broth. Press "cancel" on the Instant Pot, then turn on "multigrain" mode for 15 minutes.

While the lentils are cooking, cook the egg noodles on the stove, according to the package instructions. After the Instant Pot has finished cooking the lentils, allow the steam to release naturally. After the steam has released naturally, add the yogurt and stir. Layer the sauce on top of the noodles and garnish with fresh Italian parsley. Serve and enjoy!

Note:

If garlic is a symptom trigger, omit and use garlic-infused olive oil in the sauce. If you do not tolerate dairy, use lactose-free yogurt or a plain nut-based yogurt (such as almond yogurt).

Gluten Free, High Fiber, Fermented

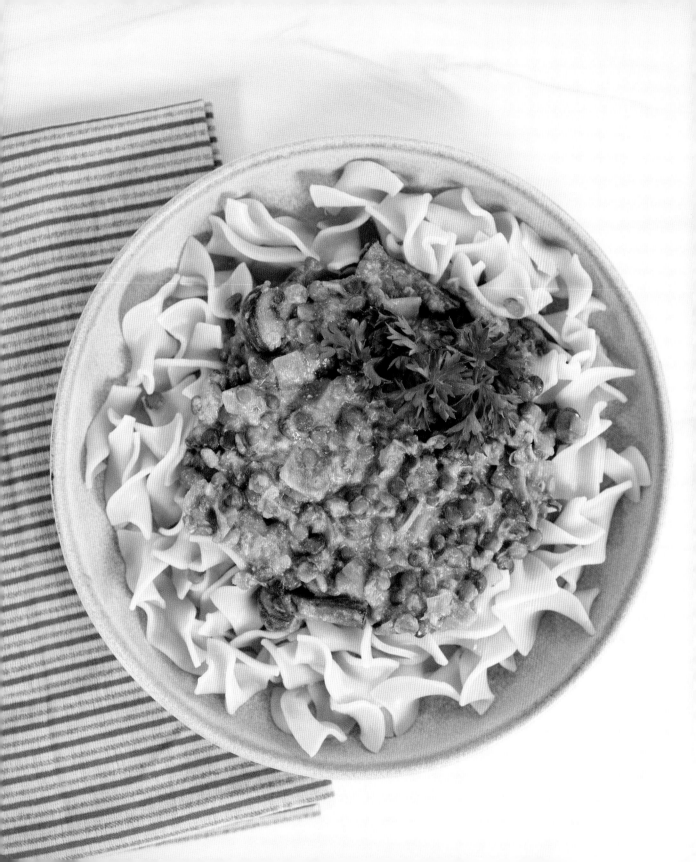

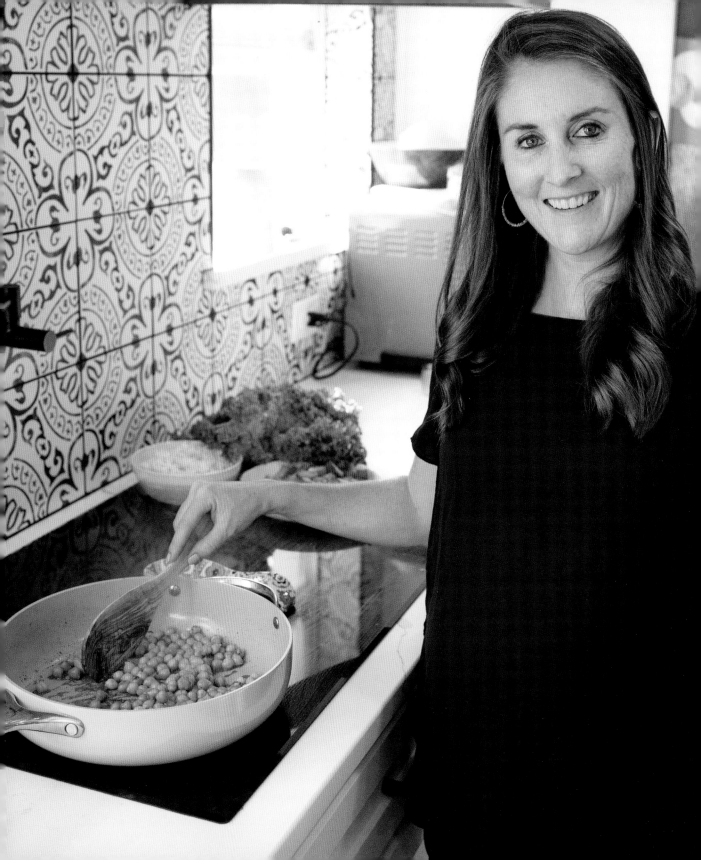

3 tbsp (45 ml) avocado oil, divided

2 purple sweet potatoes, chopped

2 tbsp (18 g) taco seasoning

1 cup (200 g) jasmine rice

2 cups (328 g) cooked chickpeas, rinsed and patted dry

2 red bell peppers, chopped

6 cups (125 g) chopped dinosaur kale

Sea salt, to taste

Black pepper, to taste

1 cup (240 ml) full-fat yogurt (I used Nancy's organic) or unsweetened coconut yogurt

Crispy Chickpeas, Sweet Potatoes and Rice

Chickpeas are added to this recipe for their fiber benefits and as an alternative to meat for protein. The soluble fiber in chickpeas fuels the good gut bacteria that can make bowel movements easier and more regular. The purple sweet potatoes are added for their antioxidant content to stimulate the growth of healthy gut bacteria including bifidobacterium and lactobacillus. The yogurt is added to provide probiotic cultures to help strengthen the digestive tract.

Makes 4 servings

Heat a skillet over medium heat. When the skillet is hot, add 1½ tablespoons (23 ml) of the avocado oil, then add the sweet potatoes. Add about half of the taco seasoning and stir to combine. Cook the sweet potato and taco seasoning mixture for 8 to 10 minutes or until the potatoes are lightly browned.

While the sweet potatoes are cooking, rinse then cook the rice according to the package instructions (or use an Instant Pot).

When the sweet potatoes are lightly browned, add the remaining 1½ tablespoons (23 ml) of the avocado oil, then add the chickpeas. Sprinkle with the remaining taco seasoning and mix to combine and cook for another 8 to 10 minutes, until the chickpeas are crispy and the sweet potatoes are soft. Add the chopped bell peppers and continue cooking while stirring for 2 more minutes. Add the kale to the skillet and cook until wilted down, 1 to 2 minutes. Add the salt and pepper to taste. Serve with rice and a dollop of yogurt!

Notes:

If you cannot tolerate kale, use any green you prefer.

If you cannot tolerate regular dairy yogurt, try lactose-free yogurt or coconut yogurt.

Gluten Free, High Fiber, Fermented

4 medium beets

1 tbsp (15 g) capers

1 cup (180 g) wild rice

½ cup (96 g) lentils

1 lemon, juiced and zested

2 tbsp (30 ml) extra virgin olive oil

1 tsp honey

¼ tsp sea salt

2 tbsp (20 g) sliced shallots

3 tbsp (21 g) raw, sprouted pumpkin seeds

¼ cup parsley (15 g), chopped (optional)

Beet and Lentil Salad with Wild Rice and Pepitas

Pumpkin seeds are added to this recipe for their high zinc content. Zinc has been shown to help improve digestive enzyme production, stomach acid production and overall immune system function. Beets and lentils are both beneficial to gut health for their high fiber content, which feeds your good gut bacteria.

Makes 2 servings

Preheat the oven to 400°F (205°C).

Wrap the beets in foil and bake for 45 to 50 minutes, or until tender when pierced. Allow the beets to cool, then rinse them under cold water. Peel the beets and chop them into quarters.

In a sauté pan over medium heat, fry the capers until just crispy, 4 to 5 minutes. You can also air fry the capers at 400°F (205°C) for 30 seconds to 1 minute.

Prepare the wild rice and the lentils according to package instructions.

In a small bowl, whisk together the lemon juice and zest, olive oil, honey and sea salt.

Add the cooked rice to a serving bowl and top with the beets, lentils, shallots and pumpkin seeds. Drizzle with the lemon dressing and top with parsley, if desired.

Notes:

To save time, use preroasted beets and precooked lentils.

To increase the protein and create a meal out of this recipe add your favorite protein, like the Roasted Lemon Chicken on page 80.

Gluten Free, Dairy Free, High Fiber

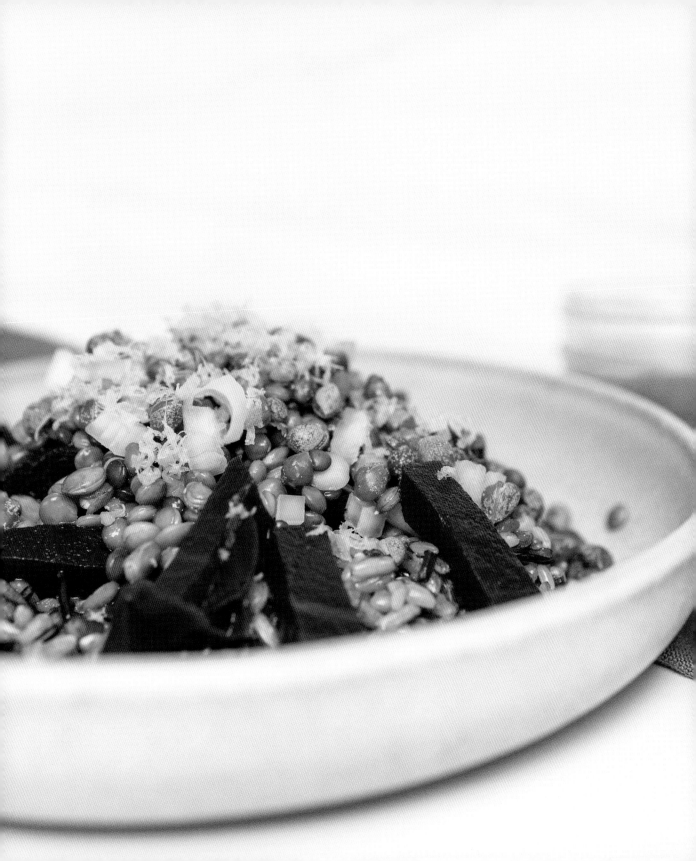

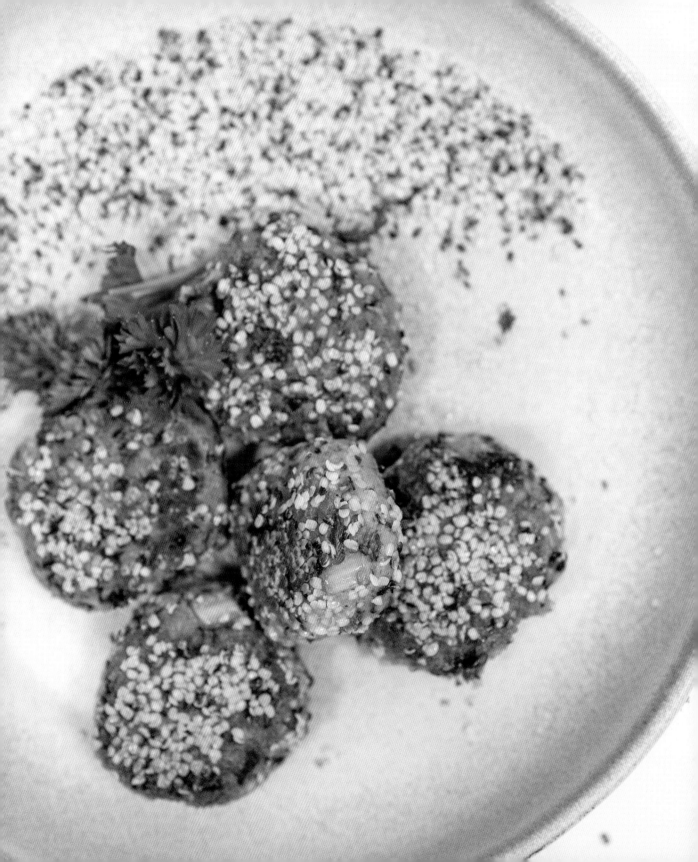

Falafels

2 tbsp (30 ml) avocado oil, divided

2 cups (136 g) chopped kale

¼ cup (15 g) flat-leaf parsley

Juice of ½ lemon

2 tsp (9 g) minced garlic

½ tsp salt

½ tsp cumin

½ tsp coriander

1 (15.5-oz [439-g]) can chickpeas

⅔ cup (132 g) cooked lentils

⅓ cup (40 g) oat flour

1 cup (160 g) hemp seeds for coating

Zesty Massaged Kale Salad

1 bunch raw kale, washed, de-stemmed and dried

¼ cup (60 ml) avocado oil

½ tsp salt

2 lemons, juiced and zested

Lemon Tahini Drizzle (page 137)

Plant-Powered Falafels with Lemon Tahini Drizzle and Zesty Massaged Kale Salad

If you love Mediterranean food as much as I do, you will love these plant-powered falafels. They are high in fiber, gluten free and so delicious. You can make these on their own or pair them with this zesty salad. The dough keeps well in the fridge for a few days if you want to make them fresh. These falafels and zesty salad have so many flavors and gut-loving ingredients, you will be satisfied from the inside out.

Makes 6 servings

In a medium pan over medium heat, add 1 tablespoon (15 ml) of the avocado oil. When the oil is hot, add the chopped kale and sauté until wilted down to about 1 cup (65 g), approximately 5 minutes.

Let the kale cool slightly, then add to a food processor along with the parsley, lemon, garlic, salt, cumin, coriander, chickpeas, lentils and oat flour. Pulse until a ball forms and the dough is sticky. The mixture will have small speckles of chickpeas and lentils but will be mostly smooth. If needed, add more lemon juice or hot water 1 tablespoon (15 ml) at a time until dough softens. Spread the hemp seeds on a small plate.

Roll the dough into 1-inch (2.5-cm) balls then roll in the hemp seeds. This will make approximately 12 balls.

Add 1 tablespoon (15 ml) of the avocado oil to a medium pan on high heat and when the oil is hot, add three to four balls to the oil. Pan-fry the balls for 4 minutes on each side on medium heat. Working in batches, repeat these steps until all the balls are cooked.

To make the salad, tear the kale into bite-sized pieces and place in a large mixing bowl. Add the avocado oil, salt and lemon juice. Massage the kale with your hands until the kale shrinks to about half its original size. Sprinkle with the lemon zest.

Serve the falafels on a bed of massaged kale with a drizzle of Lemon Tahini Drizzle. Enjoy!

Chicken and Sweet Potato Sheet Pan with Lemon Tahini Drizzle

12–14 oz (397–454 g) chicken sausage (I used Applegate Organics® chicken & apple sausage), sliced into ¼-inch (6-mm) pieces

4 sweet potatoes, chopped into 1-inch (2.5-cm) cubes

½ medium red onion, diced into chunks

8 oz (227 g) sliced baby bella mushrooms

1 lb (454 g) Brussels sprouts, bottoms trimmed, halved

3 tbsp (45 ml) avocado oil

Salt and pepper, to taste

Lemon Tahini Drizzle (page 137)

1 bunch parsley, chopped

This meal is made at least once per week in my house. It's the easiest and most delicious way to pack a lot of variety into one meal. If you are new to cooking, this is a great recipe to start with because you cannot mess it up. Swap out the veggies with what you have on hand, use different seasonings, and serve with your favorite tahini drizzle, hummus or dip. Diversity on the plate is key to a healthy gut microbiome and this meal provides nine different plants in one serving.

Makes 4 servings

Preheat the oven to 400°F (205°C).

Spread the sliced chicken sausage, sweet potatoes, onion, mushrooms and Brussels sprouts on a baking sheet. Drizzle the sausage and vegetables with the avocado oil, sprinkle with salt and pepper, then gently shake the sheet to evenly coat. Roast for 20 to 25 minutes, until the sweet potatoes are tender to the fork and chicken sausage is cooked through to 165°F (75°C).

Serve the veggies and chicken sausage with a generous amount of the Lemon Tahini Drizzle and a sprinkle of chopped parsley.

Notes:

For easier digestibility, steam the Brussels sprouts before roasting.

If you cannot tolerate onions, use leeks instead.

If you cannot tolerate garlic, use garlic-infused olive oil instead of avocado oil when making the Lemon Tahini Drizzle.

If you are short on time, skip the Lemon Tahini Drizzle and serve with store-bought tzatziki or hummus.

Gluten Free, Dairy Free, High Fiber

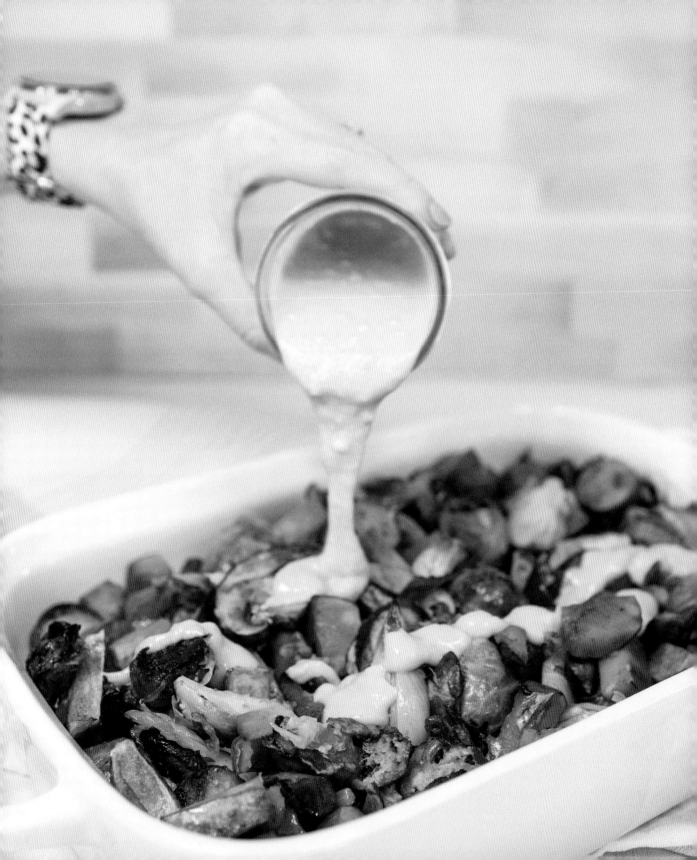

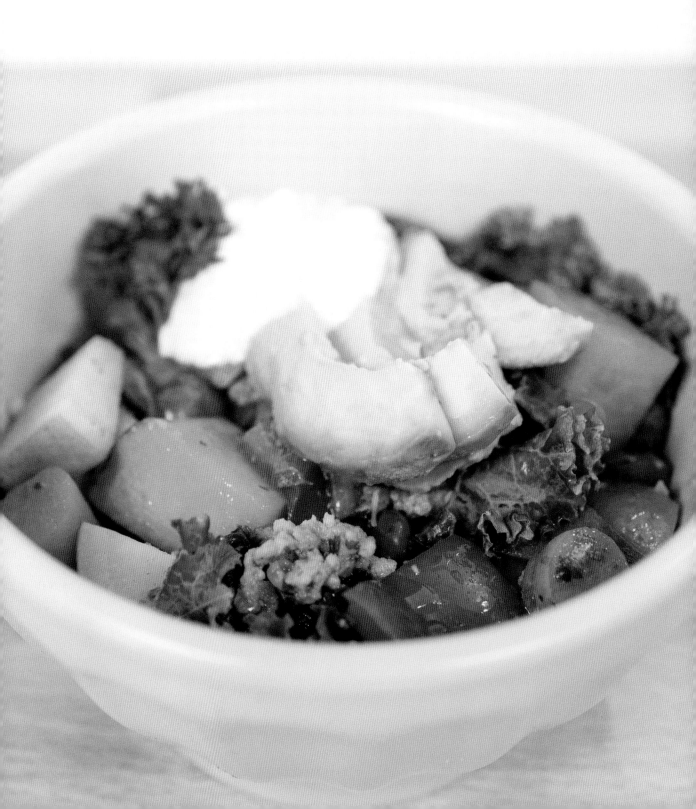

1 lb (454 g) ground beef

1 red onion, diced

2 cloves garlic, minced

2 cups (136 g) kale, destemmed and chopped

3 sweet potatoes, diced

1 red bell pepper, diced

2 carrots, diced

1 (15.5-oz [439-g]) can pinto beans, rinsed

2 cups (480 ml) beef bone broth

1 tbsp (16 g) tomato paste

2 tsp (4 g) cumin

1 tsp smoked paprika

½ tsp oregano

¼ tsp turmeric powder

½ tsp thyme

2 bay leaves

Sea salt and red pepper, to taste

Avocado, sliced, for topping

Whole-fat Greek yogurt, for topping

Slow Cooker Beef and Sweet Potato Chili

Need an easy weeknight meal that cooks while you are working? This veggie-packed chili is flavorful, full of fiber and variety and super satisfying. The best part about this recipe is that you can have everything prepped beforehand so that in the morning all you have to do is add it to the slow cooker and turn it on. Enjoy some probiotic rich full-fat yogurt when serving to add some creaminess and gut power to the top.

Makes 8 servings

Place the ground beef, onion, garlic, kale, sweet potatoes, bell pepper, carrots, pinto beans, broth, tomato paste, cumin, paprika, oregano, turmeric powder, thyme, bay leaves and salt and red pepper in a slow cooker. Cover and cook on high for 4 hours or low for 8 hours. Remove the bay leaves and serve with sliced avocado and full-fat Greek yogurt as a garnish.

Note:

Remove any ingredients that are not tolerated, or use a smaller amount.

Gluten Free, High Fiber, Fermented

Quinoa Taco Salad

½ cup (85 g) sprouted quinoa

1 cup (240 ml) Gut-Happy Broth Base (page 119) or water

2 tbsp (30 ml) avocado oil, divided

3 chicken thighs, chopped

2 limes

½ tsp cumin

½ tsp salt

Pepper, to taste

½ medium red onion, sliced

1 medium bell pepper (red or orange), chopped into ½-inch (1.3-cm) pieces

1 cup (136 g) frozen corn

1 (15.5-oz [439-g]) can black beans or equal amount of sprouted black beans

2 hearts of romaine, washed, dried and chopped

2 diced Roma tomatoes

Avocado, sliced, for topping

Mexican blend cheese (optional, use lactose-free as needed or use nutritional yeast)

1 bunch of cilantro, chopped

Greek yogurt for topping (I used Nancy's organic whole-milk Greek yogurt)

Lime Vinaigrette

¼ cup (60 ml) avocado oil

¼ tsp ground cumin

Juice of 2 limes

½ tsp salt

1 tbsp (15 ml) honey

1 tbsp (15 ml) apple cider vinegar

½ tsp yellow mustard

Pepper, to taste

Gluten Free, High Fiber

Quinoa Taco Salad with Lime Vinaigrette

Taco-bout a happy gut! This recipe is one of our go-to dinners and even easier if you prep the quinoa and the chicken in advance. For supporting gut health, this recipe is packed with fiber, color and citrus juice to help with saliva production and digestive juice secretion.

Makes 6 servings

Prepare the quinoa according to package instructions with the water or Gut-Happy Broth Base (page 119).

In a large skillet, heat 1 tablespoon (15 ml) of the avocado oil and when the oil is hot, add the chopped chicken thighs. Season the chicken with the juice of 1 lime, the cumin, salt and a sprinkle of pepper. Cook until the chicken reaches an internal temperature of 165°F (75°C), approximately 10 minutes.

In a medium skillet, sauté the red onion (if tolerated) with 1 tablespoon (15 ml) of the avocado oil on medium heat for about 2 minutes, then add the bell pepper and sauté 2 more minutes, then add the frozen corn and black beans (or sprouted beans) and stir until heated through. Squeeze the juice of the remaining lime on top of the mixture while cooking. Cook for another 5 minutes.

To make the vinaigrette, whisk or shake the avocado oil, cumin, lime juice, salt, honey, apple cider vinegar, mustard and pepper until well combined.

Assemble bowls with the romaine and Roma tomatoes, cooked quinoa and the vegetable sauté. Top with the Lime Vinaigrette, sliced avocado, cheese or nutritional yeast, cilantro, probiotic-rich Greek yogurt and additional lime wedges as desired.

Serve immediately and enjoy!

Notes:

Prep ahead: Make the quinoa, chicken and Lime Vinaigrette ahead and prepare the veggies day-of for optimal freshness.

Decrease the serving of beans to slowly introduce to your personal tolerance. For even easier digestibility, be sure to use sprouted beans (see page 157 for instructions on how to do this).

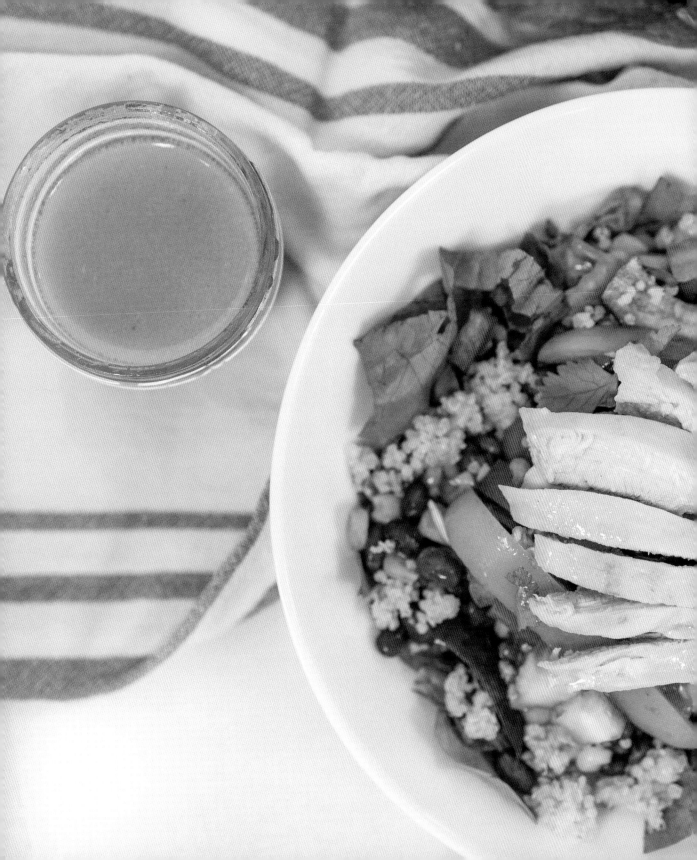

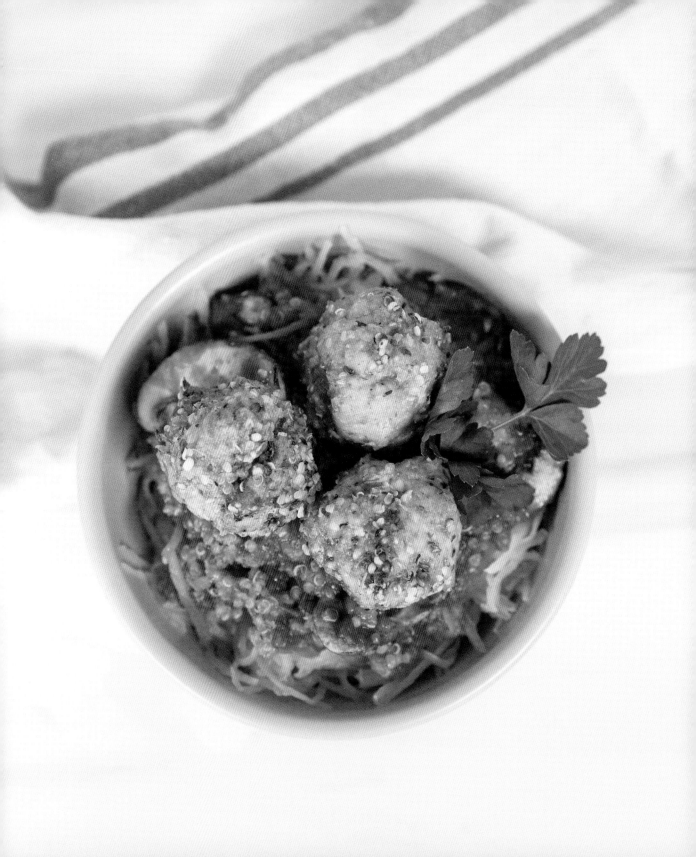

1 medium spaghetti squash

2 tbsp (30 ml) avocado oil

1 tsp salt, plus a pinch, divided

1 lb (454 g) ground turkey

½ cup (94 g) cooked quinoa, divided

6 tbsp (60 g) hemp seeds

1 tsp coconut aminos

½ tsp cumin

1½ tsp (1 g) dried parsley, divided

½ tsp pepper, divided

1½ tsp (3 g) oregano, divided

1 tbsp (15 ml) olive oil

1 cup (43 g) shredded carrots

⅛ tsp turmeric

1 tbsp (15 ml) honey

½ cup (65 g) shredded zucchini

1 cup (70 g) sliced mushrooms

1 (14.5-oz [411-g]) can chopped tomatoes

Notes:

For easier prep, cook the quinoa and spaghetti squash in advance.

Ground turkey can be replaced with ground chicken or ground beef.

For ease, you can also use canned tomato sauce (like Rao's® or Fody® for a garlic- and onion-free version).

Spaghetti Squash with Quinoa Turkey Meatballs

A fun twist on traditional spaghetti and meatballs, this recipe is loaded with fiber and flavor. This sauce is even more delicious the next day after it has had time to sit and for the flavors to marinate. Prep it in advance to enjoy throughout the week. The sauce is super flexible and so many different veggies can be added—use whatever you have on hand in your fridge!

Makes 8 servings

Preheat the oven to 400°F (205°C).

Slice a spaghetti squash in half lengthwise and remove the seeds. Drizzle the inside with avocado oil (approximately 1 tablespoon [15 ml] each side) and a pinch of salt. Pierce a few holes into the skin of the spaghetti squash and place upside-down on a baking dish. Place the spaghetti squash in the oven and cook for 30 to 40 minutes, until fork tender.

While the spaghetti squash is cooking, combine the turkey, ¼ cup (47 g) of cooked quinoa, hemp seeds, coconut aminos, cumin, ½ teaspoon of parsley, ½ teaspoon of salt, ¼ teaspoon of pepper and ½ teaspoon of oregano. Form the mixture into meatballs approximately 2 to 3 inches (5 to 8 cm) in diameter to make approximately 16 meatballs.

Place the turkey meatballs on a baking sheet and place them in the oven. Cook for 20 to 25 minutes, until cooked evenly and nicely browned.

While the meatballs are cooking, warm the olive oil over medium heat. Sauté the carrots, turmeric, honey, zucchini, ¼ teaspoon of pepper, 1 teaspoon of oregano, 1 teaspoon of parsley, ½ teaspoon of salt and the mushrooms until the mushrooms are browned, approximately 5 minutes. When the mushrooms are browned, add the canned tomatoes and remaining ¼ cup (47 g) of cooked quinoa and simmer on low for 10 minutes.

While the sauce is cooking, shred the spaghetti squash with a fork and place it in a bowl.

Serve the spaghetti squash with a generous serving of sauce and top with two or three meatballs.

Soup'er Gut
Bowls

There's nothing worse than eating a huge raw salad and feeling uncomfortably bloated afterwards. Soups are an easy way to nourish your gut with foods that are easier to digest. Switching from raw veggies to well-cooked veggies can be a great way to get the variety you love, but without the bloat. These soup recipes are great for introducing new veggies and variety and most are very easy to prepare and freeze for later. In fact, all of these soups were in my freezer for after my son was born and I was so glad to have yummy soup to heat up during the postpartum period.

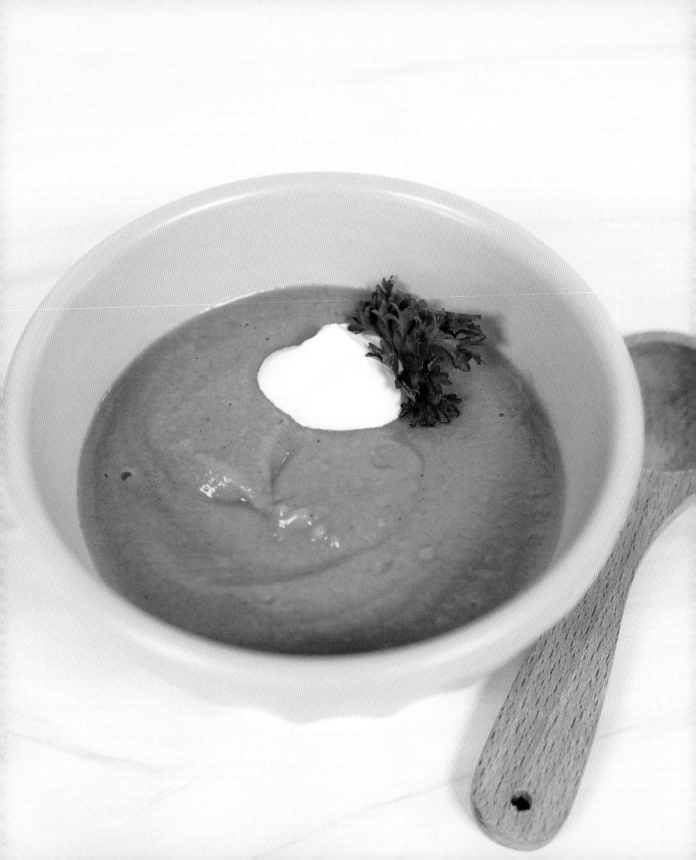

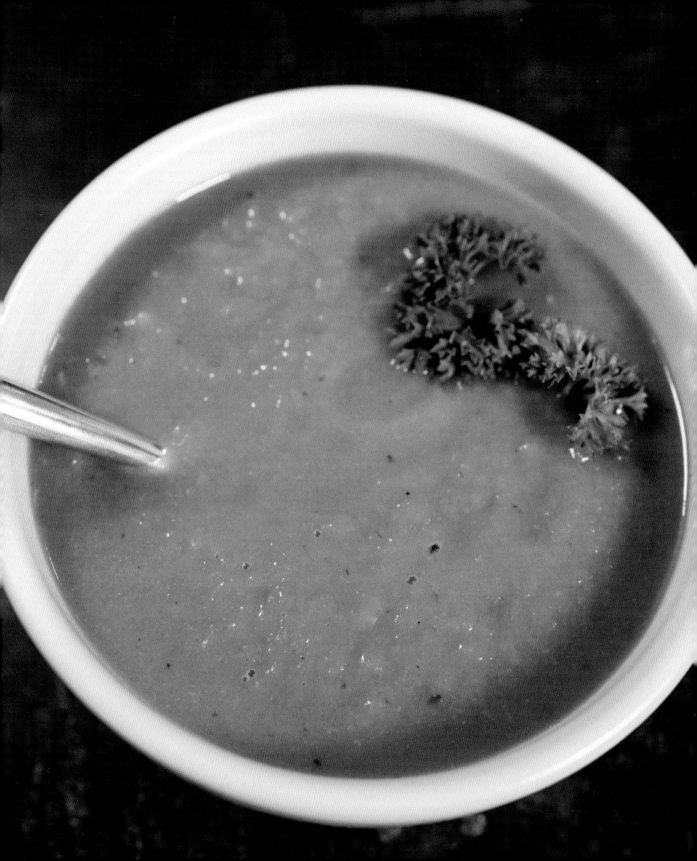

Roasted Butternut Squash and Apple Soup

1 butternut squash

Salt, to taste

1 onion

1 rib celery

1 apple (I prefer Honeycrisp)

2 tbsp (30 ml) olive oil

1 clove garlic, minced

3 tbsp (45 g) spice blend (see Notes)

2 tsp fresh grated ginger

1 tsp cayenne pepper (adjust as tolerated)

½ tsp chili powder (adjust as tolerated or omit)

6 cups (1.4 L) water or Gut-Happy Broth Base (page 119)

If you ever come to my house for dinner when it's cool outside there's a good chance this soup will be a part of the meal. It's not only delicious—but it's super easy to make and everyone loves it! This butternut squash soup is perfect for a cool evening, and the crisp apples add so much flavor and fiber. Serve this alongside your favorite protein (like the Roasted Lemon Chicken on page 80) or as an appetizer with some toasty sourdough for dipping.

Makes 6 servings

Preheat the oven to 350°F (175°C).

Cut the butternut squash in half and sprinkle sea salt on top of each half. Roast the squash on a baking sheet for 1 hour or until the squash is fork tender. Cube the squash while still hot (I leave the skin on, but you can remove it if you prefer).

While the butternut squash is cooking, dice the onion and celery into small pieces. Core the apple and then dice into chunks (I left the skin on for extra fiber but you can remove if you prefer).

In a large pot over medium heat, warm the olive oil. Sauté the onion, celery, garlic, spice blend, ginger, cayenne and chili powder until caramelized, 3 to 5 minutes. When the mixture is caramelized, add the water or broth and roasted butternut squash and apple cubes. Simmer for approximately 20 minutes or until all ingredients are soft. Puree the soup with a hand blender until it is smooth with no chunks. Serve and enjoy!

Notes:

- For the spice blend, I used Trader Joe's® 21 Seasoning Salute, but to make your own, mix ½ teaspoon each of parsley and oregano, ¼ teaspoon each of pepper, rosemary, garlic, basil, celery seed, cayenne pepper, thyme and cumin, and 1 bay leaf.

- Remove any spices that are not tolerated or use smaller amounts.

- Use less apple if not tolerated or substitute with 2 chopped carrots.

Gluten Free, Dairy Free, High Fiber, Vegan

2 tbsp (30 ml) avocado oil

1 medium yellow onion, diced

1 tsp garlic, minced

1 (1-inch [2.5-cm]) knob ginger, zested

6 cups (768 g) chopped carrots (from approximately 6 large carrots)

10 cups (2.4 L) vegetable broth or Gut-Happy Broth Base (see Note)

3 cups (300 g) cooked farro

Nutty Ginger and Carrot Soup

If you've never cooked with farro, you are missing out. This nutty grain is high in fiber, really filling and satisfying with the creaminess of the carrot soup. The fiber in the carrots and the ginger will leave your gut not only feeling satisfied but also will help reduce symptoms and eliminate bloat.

Enjoy this alongside your favorite protein side for a balanced meal.

Makes 4 servings

To make this on the stove, combine the avocado oil, onion, garlic, ginger and carrots in a medium pan over medium heat. Cook until the onions are translucent and the carrots are a little soft, approximately 5 minutes. Add the broth and bring to a boil. Cover and simmer until the carrots are soft and cooked through, approximately 10 minutes. Let the soup cool slightly, then add it to a blender and puree until smooth (or use an immersion blender inside the pot). Transfer the soup back to the pot and add the farro. Bring the soup back to a boil and cook for 10 more minutes.

To make this in an Instant Pot, on sauté mode combine the onion, garlic, ginger and carrots in avocado oil. Cook until the onions are translucent and the carrots are mildly soft, approximately 5 minutes. Add the broth and cook on manual high pressure for 15 minutes then let the pressure manually release. Let the soup cool slightly, then add to a blender and puree until smooth (or use an immersion blender inside of the Instant Pot). Transfer the soup back to the Instant Pot and add the farro. Cook on manual high pressure for 13 minutes.

Note:

If you use the Gut-Happy Broth Base on page 119, this recipe will no longer be vegan.

Dairy Free, High Fiber, Vegan

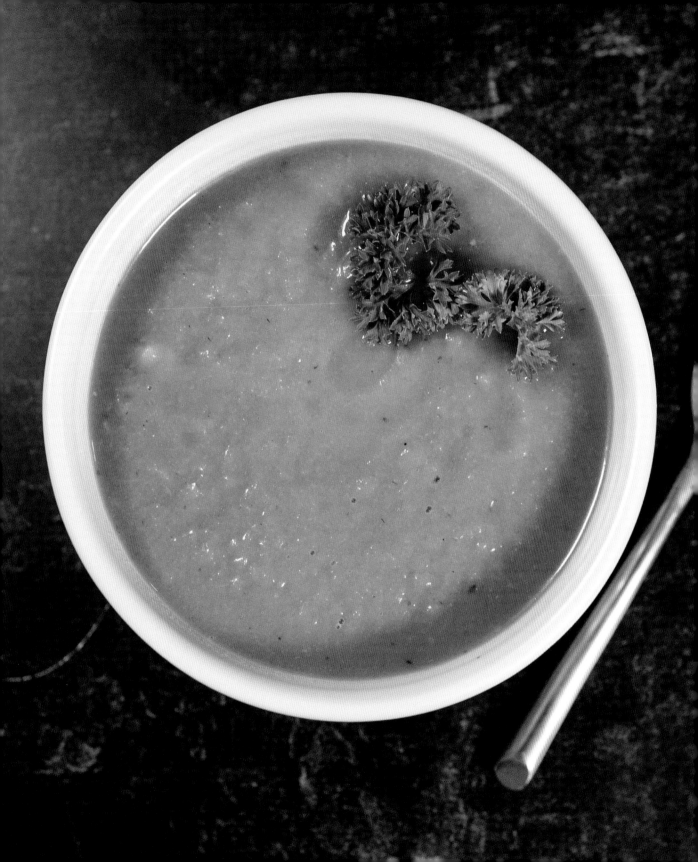

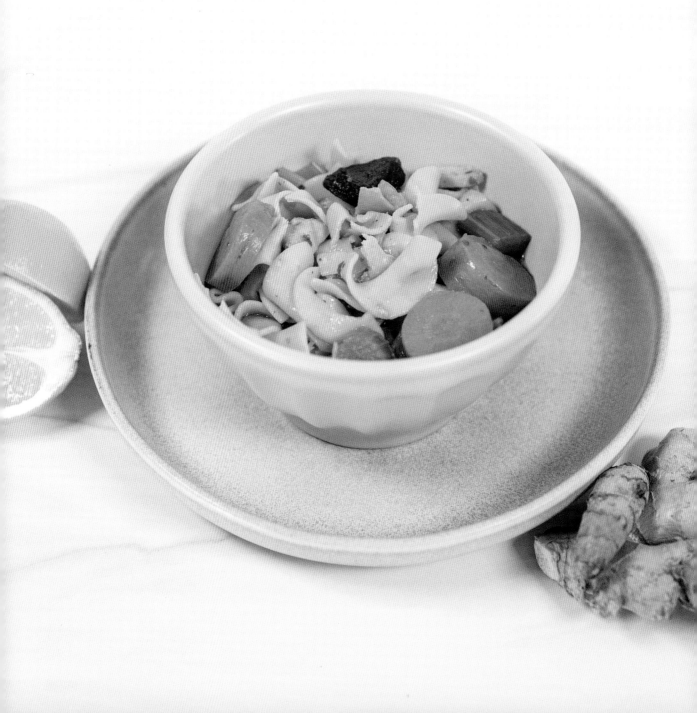

1 medium red onion, diced

1 tsp minced garlic

1 tsp minced ginger

1 tsp grated fresh turmeric

1 tbsp (15 ml) avocado oil

3 ribs celery, sliced

2 carrots, sliced

½ tsp salt

1 tsp dried oregano

1 tsp dried parsley

2 cups (145 g) sliced cremini mushrooms

10 cups (2.4 L) chicken bone broth or Gut-Happy Broth Base (page 119)

1 lb (454 g) chicken thighs

1 sprig fresh rosemary

3 cups (360 g) egg noodles

4 lemons

Happy Gut Chicken Soup

This recipe is one of my favorites, especially with the added lemon flavor. It is so satisfying and a recipe we make on repeat in my house, especially in the wintertime. This is also a great soup to prepare and freeze for when you need it most. It not only contains super mineral-rich broth for your gut, but also contains lots of anti-inflammatory spices for soothing your gut. Trust me, don't skip the lemon on top!

Makes 8 servings

In a soup pot over medium heat, sauté the onion, garlic, ginger, turmeric and avocado oil until the onion is translucent, approximately 5 minutes. Add the celery, carrots, salt, oregano, parsley and mushrooms and sauté on medium heat for 5 minutes.

Add the broth, chicken and rosemary to the pot and bring to a boil. Simmer for 20 minutes or until the chicken is cooked through to 165°F (75°C).

Remove the chicken from the pot and when it is slightly cooled, shred it by hand or with two forks. While you are shredding the chicken, add the egg noodles to the pot and simmer, uncovered, for 8 to 10 minutes until the egg noodles are cooked. Return the shredded chicken to the pot and let it warm through.

Serve with a squeeze of half of a lemon on top of each bowl.

Gluten Free, Dairy Free

1 tbsp (15 ml) avocado oil

1 red onion, diced

1 tsp minced garlic

1 tsp minced ginger

¾ tsp salt

1 tsp minced fresh turmeric (or ground)

2 medium sweet potatoes, chopped into 1-inch (2.5-cm) cubes

1 red bell pepper, chopped into 1-inch (2.5-cm) cubes

1 (15.5-oz [439-g]) can white northern beans

2 cups (480 ml) chicken or Gut-Happy Broth Base (page 119)

Juice of ½ lemon

Creamy Sweet Potato Soup

This delicious soup contains the secret ingredient of white beans to add creaminess, flavor and fiber. Sweet potatoes and white beans are both rich in fiber and when this soup is prepared and stored, it also will become a source of resistant starch to further fuel your gut bacteria. In addition to the fiber, sweet potatoes are also a rich source of anti-oxidants and vitamins to keep your gut and body happy and healthy.

Makes 6 servings

To make this on the stove: in a soup pot over medium heat, warm the avocado oil then sauté the onion, garlic, ginger, salt and turmeric until fragrant, about 3 minutes. Add the sweet potatoes and bell pepper and continue to sauté until the sweet potatoes are slightly browned on the outside, about 5 minutes. Add the white beans and chicken broth or Gut-Happy Broth Base and bring the mixture to a boil. Cover and simmer until the sweet potatoes are fork tender. Squeeze lemon juice on top of the soup and stir it until completely combined. Enjoy!

To make this in an Instant Pot: on sauté mode, combine the avocado oil, onion, garlic, ginger, salt and turmeric and cook until fragrant, about 3 minutes. Add the sweet potatoes and bell pepper and continue to sauté until the sweet potatoes are slightly browned on the outside, about 5 minutes. Add the white beans and chicken broth or Gut-Happy Broth Base and cover with the Instant Pot lid. Cook on manual high-pressure mode for 15 minutes, then let the steam naturally release. Squeeze lemon juice on top of the soup and stir it until completely combined. Enjoy!

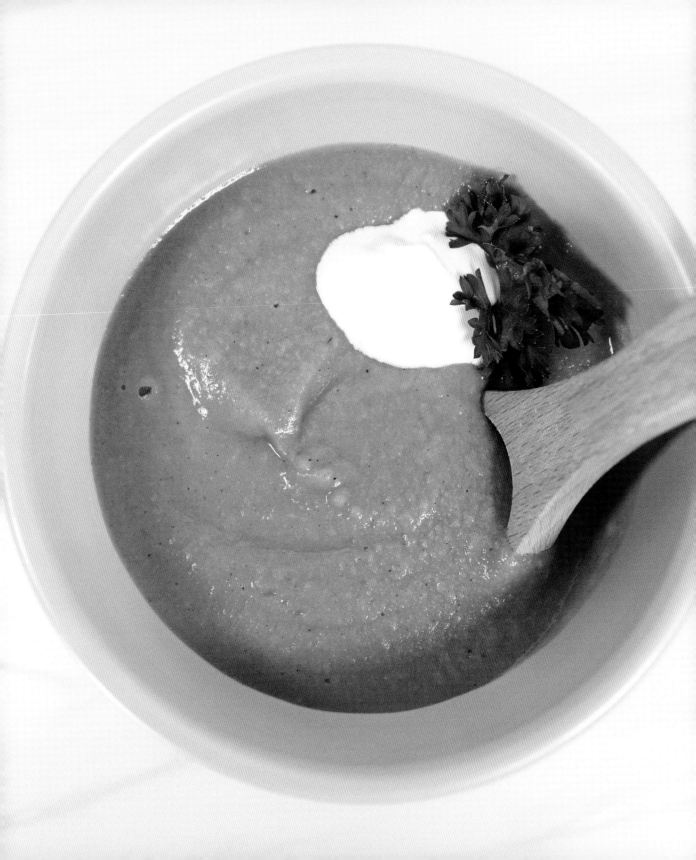

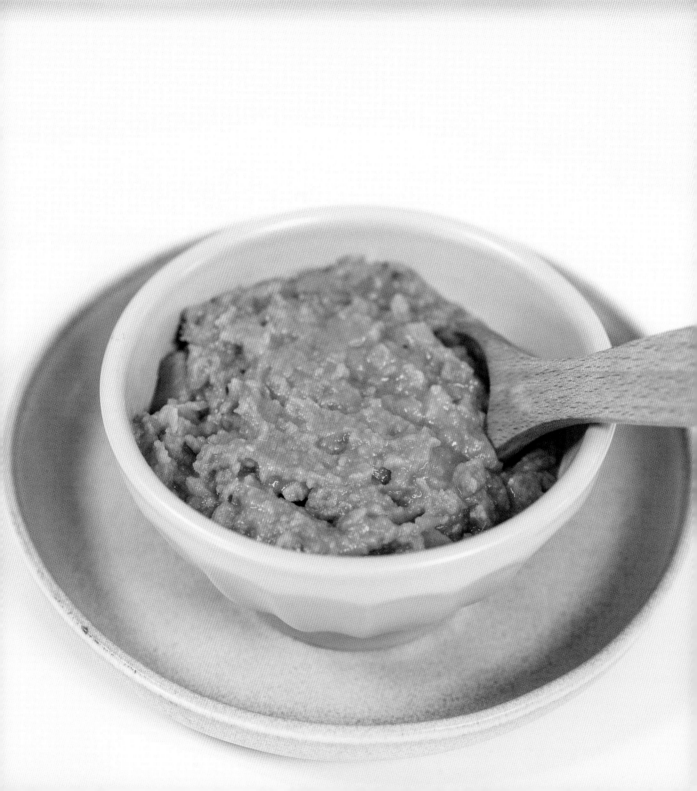

2 tbsp (30 ml) avocado oil

1 yellow onion, chopped

1 yellow bell pepper, chopped

½ tsp salt

2 cups (345 g) white baby potatoes, halved

1 lb (454 g) dried split peas

1 qt (960 ml) chicken bone broth

Split Pea Soup

This soup puts a spin on traditional split pea soup with the addition of baby potatoes. When cooked and cooled, baby potatoes are an excellent source of resistant starch, which acts like a prebiotic to feed good gut bacteria. In addition, split peas are an excellent source of soluble fiber—the exact fiber we want to help feed our good gut bacteria. Split peas are also an excellent source of iron, zinc, protein and phosphorous. After a big bowl of this soup your gut bacteria is sure to be satisfied!

Makes 6 servings

To make this on the stove: in a soup pot over medium heat, warm the avocado oil then add the onion and bell pepper. Sprinkle with the salt and cook until the onion is translucent, approximately 5 minutes. Add the halved potatoes, split peas and bone broth. Cover and simmer until the potatoes and split peas are tender, about 30 minutes. Puree in a blender or with an immersion blender and serve.

To make this in an Instant Pot: on sauté mode, add the oil and heat. When the oil is hot add the onion, bell pepper and salt. Cook for 10 minutes or until the vegetables are soft. Add the halved potatoes, split peas and bone broth. Cook on manual mode, high pressure for 15 minutes. Let the soup cool slightly and add to a blender and puree until smooth or desired consistency.

Gluten Free, Dairy Free, High Fiber

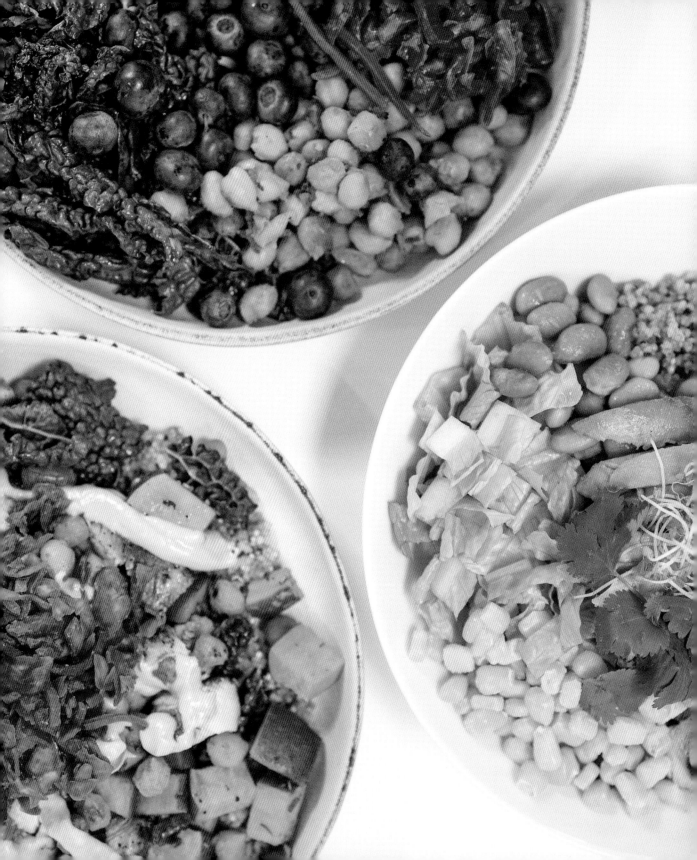

Biome Bowls

Prepping ahead and having food prepared can create less stress for both you and your gut. One of the easiest ways to get in plant diversity throughout the week is in the form of easy-to-make biome bowls. Prep the ingredients, switch up the toppings and dressings and you have a diverse and delicious bowl for a quick and easy meal.

The basic outline for a biome bowl is to include protein, fat, fibrous carbs, color, fermented flavor and if desired, a sauce. You can keep the same structure for each bowl, but switch out what goes into each food category as the week goes on.

For ease, I choose at least one day of the week to prep some easy proteins, beans, grains and sauces so that my meals throughout the week (especially lunches) are simple, yet delicious and fiber filled. Incorporating some form of meal prep (even just 30 minutes on a Sunday) can save you stress and time throughout the week. Trust me, your gut will thank you!

Protein	Fat	Fibrous Carbs	Color	Fermented Flavor	Sauce
Chicken	Avocado	Quinoa	Kale	Pickled Beets (page 149)	Kefir Tzatziki (page 149)
Salmon	Classic Hummus (page 134)	Brown rice	Arugula	Sauerkraut (page 148)	Olive oil
Beef	Lemon Tahini Drizzle (page 137)	Farro	Green beans	Kefir (page 147)	Cilantro-Lime (page 137)
Tuna	Olives	Potatoes	Romaine	Probiotic-rich yogurt	Barbecue Sauce (page 137)
Crispy Chickpeas (page 89)	Olive oil	Carrots	Chard	Pickles	Fresh Herb Dressing (page 137)
Tofu	Pesto (see page 140 for recipes)	Sweet potatoes	Spinach	Olives	Teriyaki Dressing (page 137)
Tempeh	Nuts	Buckwheat	Zesty Massaged Kale Salad (page 93)	Cheese	Lemon Tahini Drizzle (page 137)
Natto	Feta	Beans/chickpeas	Crispy Honey Lime Brussels Sprouts (page 82)	Kimchi	Classic Hummus (page 134)
Nutritional Yeast	Goat cheese	Teff	Cabbage	Miso	Vinegar

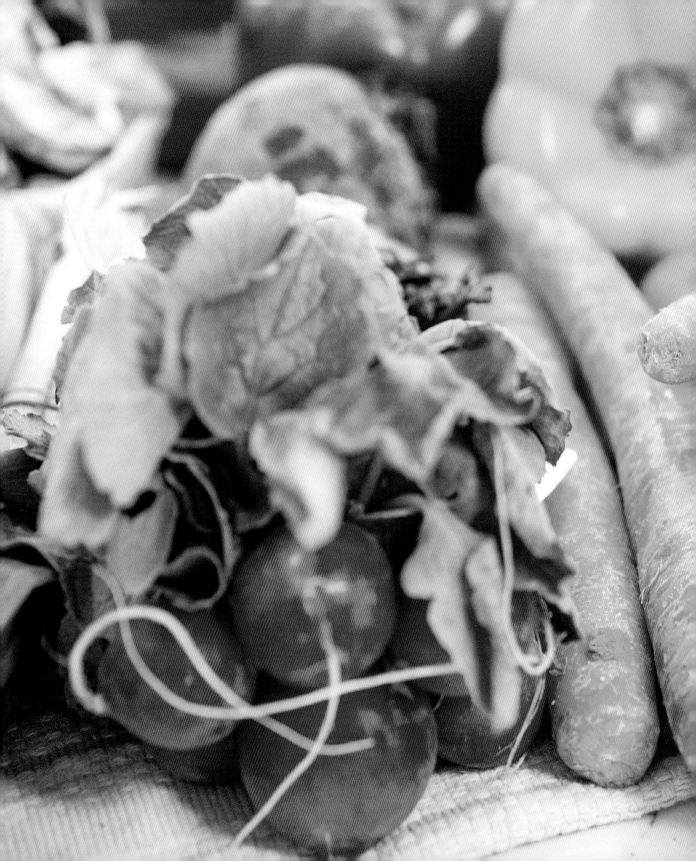

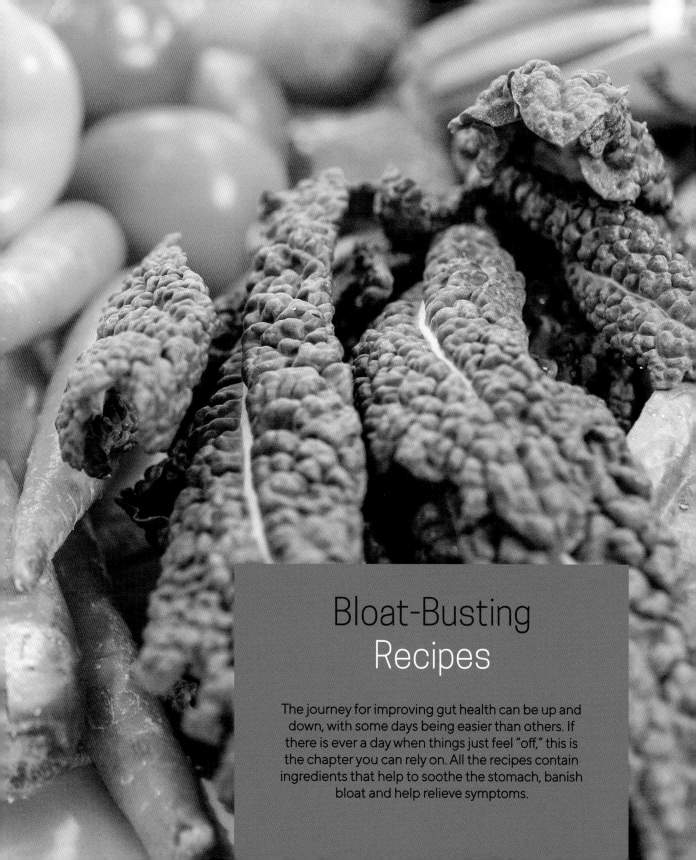

Bloat-Busting Recipes

The journey for improving gut health can be up and down, with some days being easier than others. If there is ever a day when things just feel "off," this is the chapter you can rely on. All the recipes contain ingredients that help to soothe the stomach, banish bloat and help relieve symptoms.

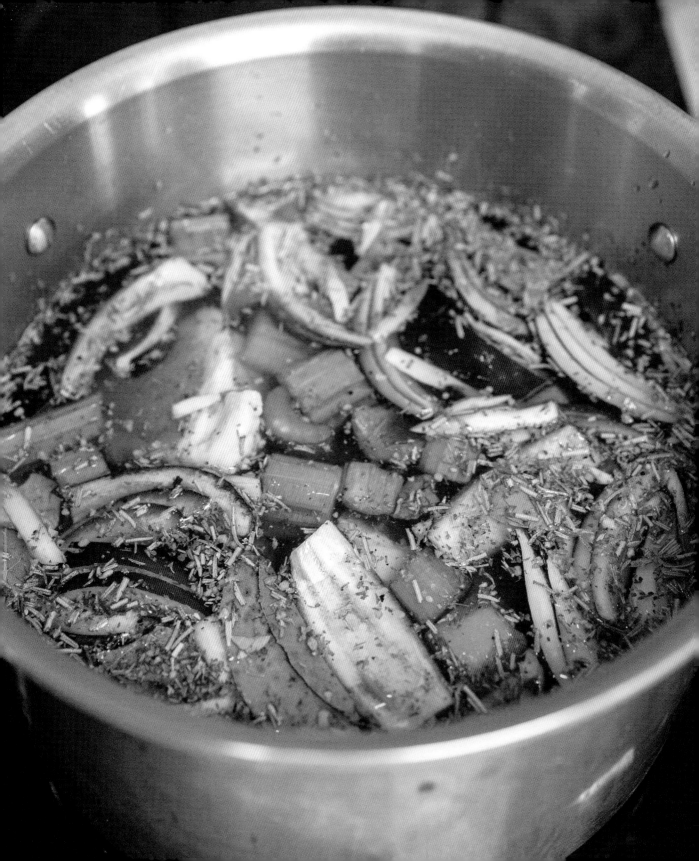

About 3 lb (1.4 kg) chicken or beef bones (I like to use the marrow)

Water to cover the bones by 2 inches (5 cm)

1 onion, chopped into large chunks

3 carrots, chopped

3 ribs celery, chopped

1 potato, diced

1 tbsp (15 ml) apple cider vinegar

1 tbsp (18 g) sea salt

4 bay leaves

2 tsp (3 g) herbs de Provence (optional)

Gut-Happy Broth Base

This super nourishing broth is a great base for any soup that you are making or even by itself with some sliced avocado and squeezed lemon. You can also use this broth as a base for cooking grains like quinoa, rice or farro. This broth is rich in minerals, collagen, fat and protein.

Makes about 3 quarts (2.8 L)

To make this in a slow cooker, add all the ingredients to a slow cooker. Make sure there is at least 1 inch (2.5 cm) of space from the lid. Secure the slow cooker lid and cook on low for 24 hours. Strain the broth into a bowl to remove the vegetables, bones and bay leaves.

To make this in an Instant Pot, add all the ingredients and put the Instant Pot on manual mode and set the timer for 90 minutes. When it is done cooking allow the pressure to release for 10 to 15 minutes before quick-releasing the steam (or let it fully release on its own). Strain the broth into a bowl to remove the vegetables, bones and bay leaves.

Freeze the broth in large mason jars or freeze small amounts in a cupcake pan for single servings.

Notes:

- You can find bones at your local farmers' market, in the freezer section of some grocery stores or from buying your chicken whole and saving the bones after you use the meat (buy an organic chicken).

- This broth will last 5 to 6 days in the fridge or for 2 to 3 months in the freezer.

Gluten Free, Dairy Free

2 cups (480 ml) unsweetened almond milk or full-fat coconut milk

1 date

½ tsp turmeric

¼ tsp ginger

⅛ tsp cinnamon

⅛ tsp cardamom

⅛ tsp cloves

Pinch of black pepper

1 tbsp (10 g) collagen protein

Gutsy Golden Milk

This hot and warming drink is like a hug in a cup. When you are feeling off or if your stomach is just not right, this hot cup of sunshine is sure to ease some of your digestive woes. Made with anti-inflammatory herbs and spices, this is an all-around win for your gut.

Makes 1 serving

Heat the almond milk in the microwave on high for 90 seconds (or until desired temperature) or on the stove. Add the warmed almond milk, date, turmeric, ginger, cinnamon, cardamom, cloves, black pepper and collagen protein to a blender and blend for approximately 1 minute on medium speed. Be sure to leave a crack in the lid for any steam to escape. Pour into a big mug and enjoy!

Gluten Free, Dairy Free

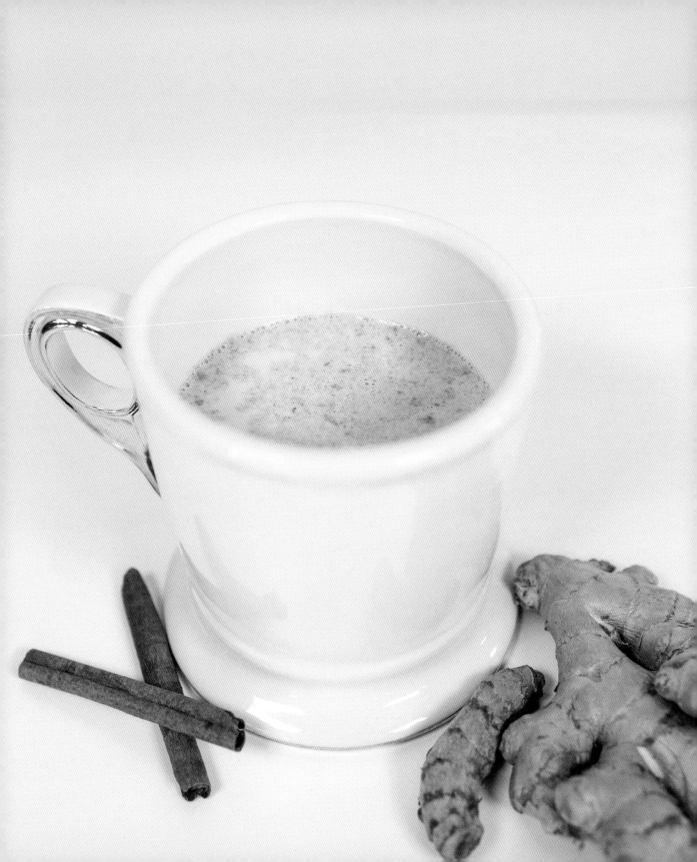

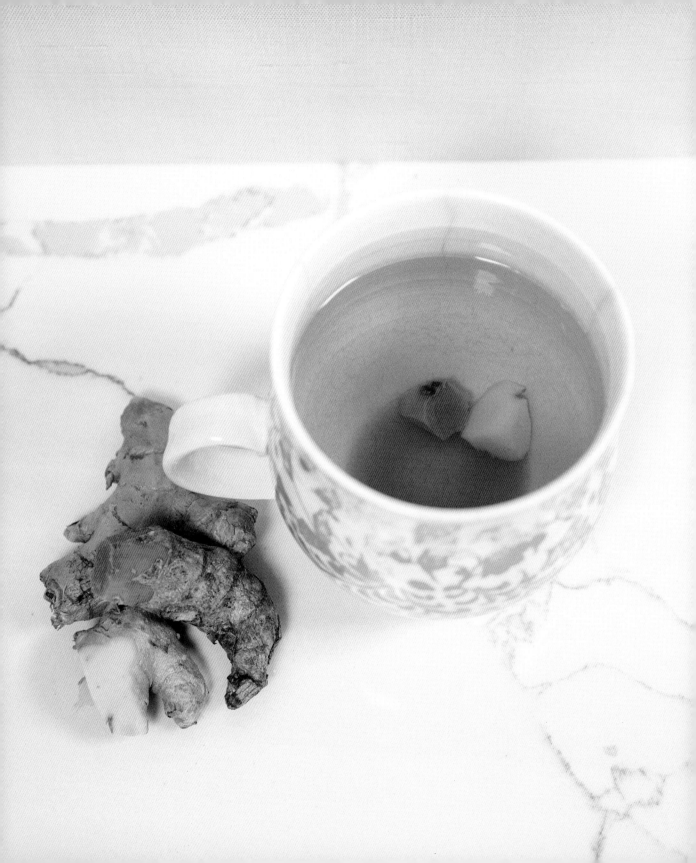

1 cup (240 ml) water

¼-inch (6-mm) slice fresh ginger

¼-inch (6-mm) slice fresh turmeric

½ lemon, squeezed

Honey (optional)

Happy Digestion Tea

Both turmeric and ginger are soothing to the gut and great for times when your stomach just feels "off." Ginger is helpful at improving gut motility (the movement of the gut muscles) and turmeric helps to calm down any inflammation. Together, these herbs are soothing to the gut and can help relieve bloating, constipation, gas and diarrhea.

Makes 1 serving

Bring the water to a boil. Scrape the edge of a spoon against the fresh ginger root to remove the skin. Use a vegetable peeler to remove the skin from the fresh turmeric root. Place the ginger and turmeric slices in a mug and pour the boiling water on top. Add the lemon juice. Steep for 10 to 15 minutes then remove the ginger and turmeric knobs. Add honey if desired.

Gluten Free, Dairy Free, Vegan

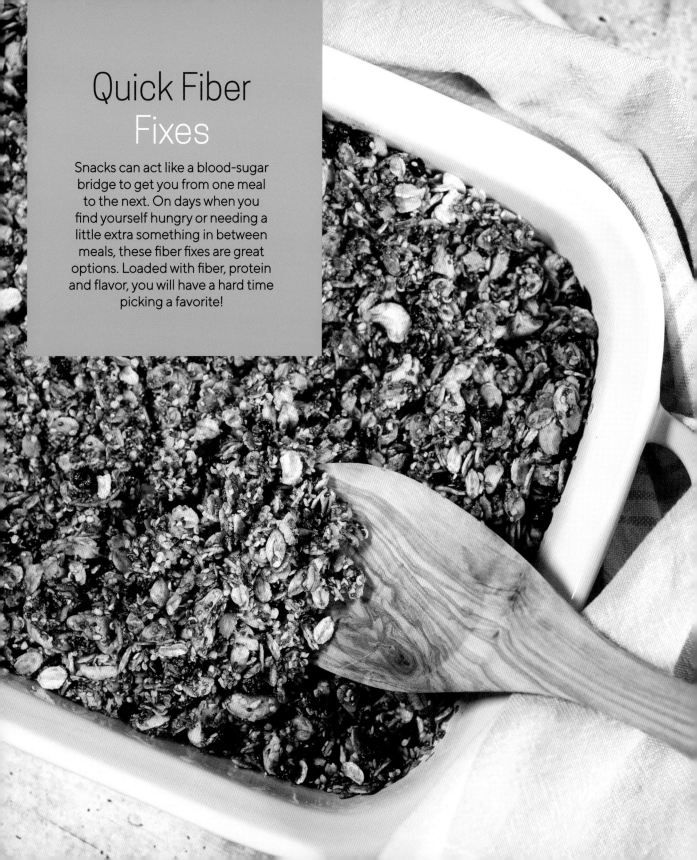

Quick Fiber Fixes

Snacks can act like a blood-sugar bridge to get you from one meal to the next. On days when you find yourself hungry or needing a little extra something in between meals, these fiber fixes are great options. Loaded with fiber, protein and flavor, you will have a hard time picking a favorite!

Cashew Crunch High Fiber Granola

1½ cups (125 g) gluten free rolled oats

½ cup (56 g) cashew pieces (or any nut you like)

½ cup (48 g) coconut flakes

½ cup (88 g) chia seeds

⅓ cup (53 g) hemp seeds

½ cup (60 g) dried blueberries

⅓ cup (80 ml) honey (or maple syrup)

2 tbsp (30 ml) coconut oil

½ tsp cinnamon

1 tsp vanilla extract

Pinch of salt

Granola is one of my favorite additions to any smoothie bowl, yogurt parfait, chia pudding or overnight oats recipe. This fiber-filled recipe is satisfying to your gut and has just enough crunch to add texture and flavor to any meal. This recipe is super flexible, so if you prefer another nut to cashews, feel free to swap. You can also easily double the recipe and have more to share!

Makes ten ½-cup (50-g) servings

Preheat the oven to 325°F (165°C).

In a bowl, combine the oats, cashews, coconut flakes, chia seeds, hemp seeds and dried blueberries. Set aside.

In a small saucepan over low heat, combine the honey or maple syrup, coconut oil and cinnamon until everything is melted. Remove the pan from the heat and stir in the vanilla and salt.

Mix the honey mixture with the granola until well coated.

Transfer the granola to two baking sheets and place in the oven. Bake the granola for 15 minutes and then rotate the pans to continue to bake the granola for another 15 minutes. You want the granola to be golden brown, so continue rotating the pans if it isn't golden at the 30-minute mark. Avoid stirring the granola if you want clusters!

Allow the granola to cool before transferring to an airtight container. Eat as a snack or top your favorite parfait, oatmeal or chia pudding with this crunchy treat!

Gluten Free, Dairy Free, High Fiber

½ cup (120 ml) raw, unfiltered honey

½ cup (128 g) natural almond butter

2 tbsp (30 ml) coconut oil

1 tsp pure vanilla extract

2 tbsp (16 g) cinnamon

¾ cup (75 g) raw pecan halves

¾ cup (90 g) raw walnuts

½ cup (70 g) raw almonds

5 large pitted dates, soaked in warm water for 15 minutes

¼ cup (20 g) shredded, unsweetened coconut

¼ cup (35 g) raisins (optional)

¼ cup (30 g) dried blueberries or cranberries (optional)

½ cup (120 g) dark chocolate chunks or chips (optional)

Cinna-Brain Bars

This was one of the first recipes I ever developed and is still one of my favorite snacks to have on hand. These bars are packed with gut- and brain-loving ingredients that will leave you satisfied and are a great bridge between meals. These bars promote brain health by providing omega-3 fatty acids (walnuts) and medium chain fatty acids (coconut oil). They are anti-inflammatory, and an excellent source of antioxidants. The phenylethylamine (PEA) in dark chocolate encourages the brain to release endorphins, and increases the blood flow to the brain, therefore improving cognitive function.

Makes 12 servings

Line an 8 x 8–inch (20 x 20–cm) pan with parchment paper.

Place the honey, almond butter, coconut oil, vanilla and cinnamon in a saucepan over medium heat. Bring to a boil, then lower the heat and simmer for 15 minutes.

Meanwhile, place the pecans, walnuts, almonds and dates in a food processor and process until the mixture resembles coarse sand. Add the coconut and pulse a few times to combine.

Remove the honey mixture from the stove, and stir in the nut mixture. Let the mixture cool, then add the raisins, dried berries and dark chocolate, if desired. Spoon the mixture into the parchment-lined baking dish, and use a large piece of parchment paper to help you press the mixture evenly across the pan. Pack tightly.

Remove the parchment paper and place the dish in the freezer for 2 hours. Remove from the freezer and cut evenly into 12 rectangular bars. Store the bars in the refrigerator in an airtight container.

Notes:

If you prefer, use maple syrup instead of honey.

Use any dried fruit you prefer to change the flavor slightly (like dried apricots, etc.).

All nuts could be swapped for seeds such as pumpkin, sunflower or sesame seeds.

Gluten Free, Dairy Free, High Fiber

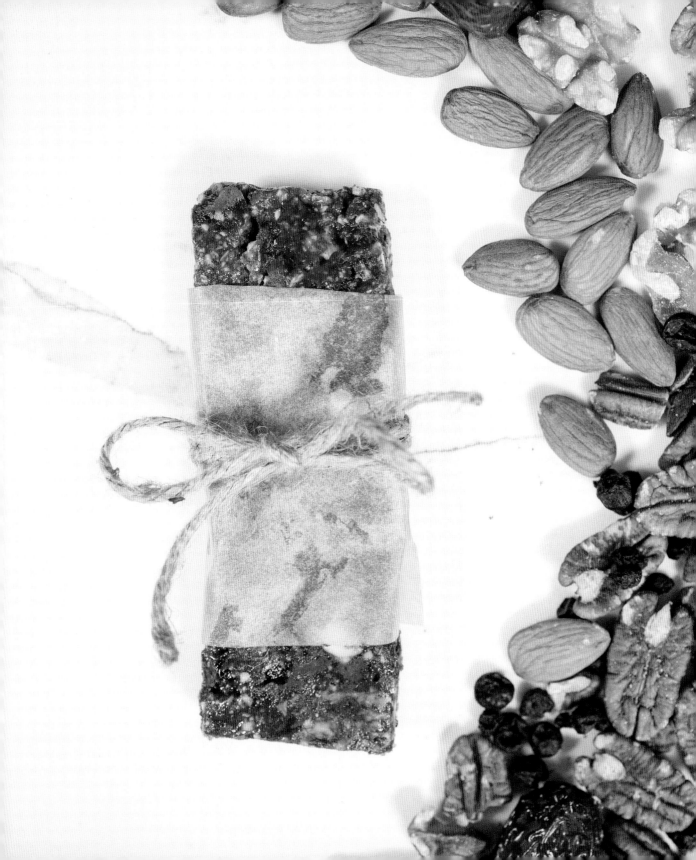

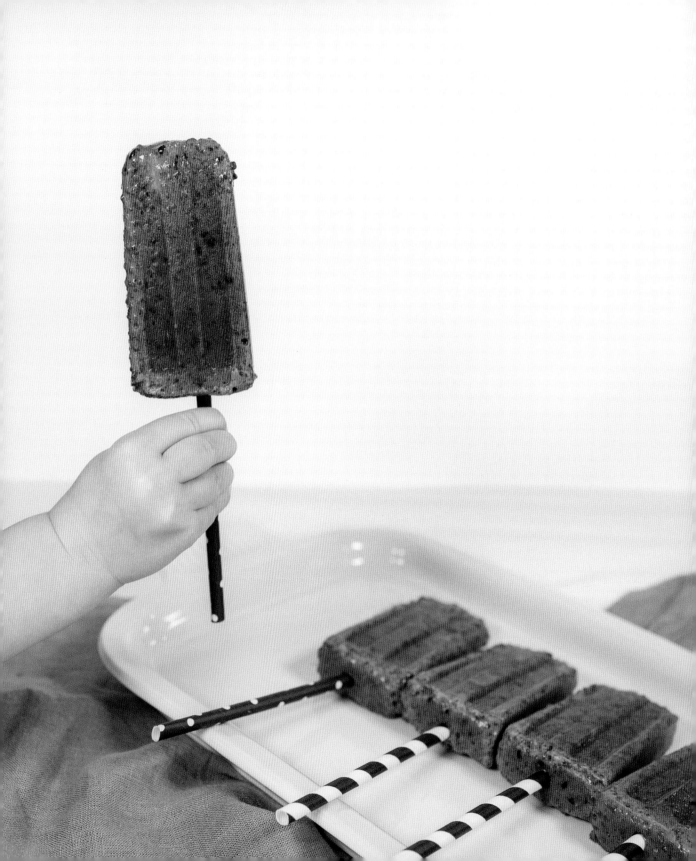

3 cups (560 g) frozen berries

2 cups (480 ml) plain Kefir
(page 147; or almond milk)

1 banana, frozen

¼ cup (44 g) chia seeds

¼ cup (40 g) collagen powder
(or unflavored protein powder)

Probiotic Fruit Pops

Are you in need of a refreshing summer snack? These probiotic fruit pops are a satisfying, protein- and fiber-filled snack that will not only taste refreshing but also make your gut super happy. My daughter loves these popsicles on a hot day in the summer or even for a fun breakfast!

Makes 4 servings

Place all the ingredients in a blender and blend until smooth. Pour into popsicle molds and freeze for at least 4 hours! Enjoy!

Note:

If you cannot tolerate kefir, add 1 tablespoon (15 ml) at a time (filling in the rest of the liquid with almond milk) or use a quarter to half of the amount of kefir as your body adjusts.

Gluten Free, High Fiber, Fermented

Pumpkin Cacao Fiber Bites

10 Medjool dates

1½ cups (155 g) sprouted oats

½ cup (129 g) peanut butter or almond butter

½ cup (120 ml) pumpkin puree (not pie filling)

¼ cup (44 g) chia seeds

¼ cup (40 g) flaxseeds

1 tsp vanilla extract

1 tsp ground cinnamon

¼ tsp ground ginger

¼ tsp ground nutmeg

¼ tsp salt

3 tbsp (45 g) dark chocolate chips

Cacao powder, for dusting

Want to enjoy fall flavors all year long? These pumpkin fiber bites are a little slice of fall, wrapped with fiber and gut-loving ingredients. These fiber bites are great to have on hand for a quick snack, breakfast addition or even a sweet bite after a meal. Easy to make and store, these are a convenient meal prep option that your gut and family will love.

Makes 12 servings

Soak the dates in hot water for 10 minutes. After soaking, easily remove the seeds and throw away (if your dates do not have seeds, you can skip this step).

Add the soaked dates to a food processor along with the sprouted oats, peanut or almond butter, pumpkin puree, chia seeds, flaxseeds, vanilla, cinnamon, ginger, nutmeg and salt and process until smooth. The mixture will be thick and sticky. If it is too sticky and difficult to blend, add hot water, 1 tablespoon (15 ml) at a time, until it blends into a very sticky ball.

Transfer the sticky ball to a large bowl and mix in the chocolate chips. Roll the mixture into 1-inch (2.5-cm) balls and dust the balls generously with cacao powder. Store in the fridge in an airtight container for up to 7 days.

Gluten Free, Dairy Free, High Fiber, Vegan

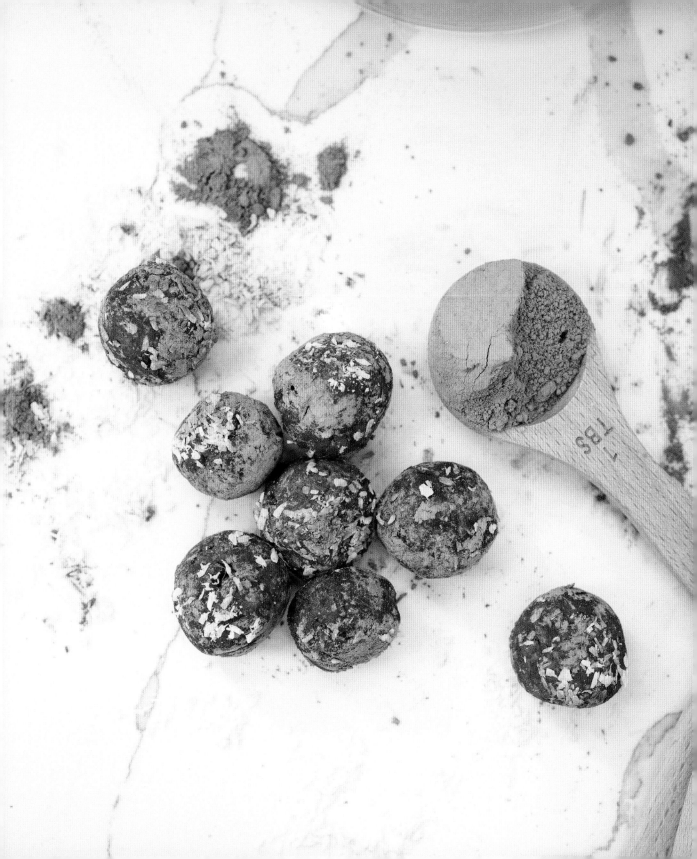

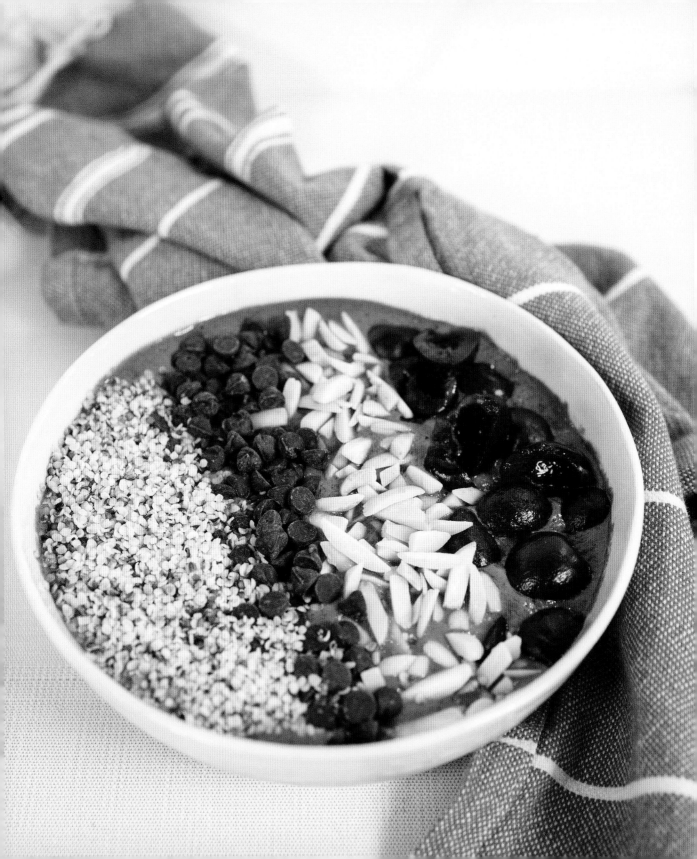

2 cups (310 g) frozen cherries

½ cup (120 ml) unsweetened almond milk

½ cup (120 ml) Kefir (page 147; use goat's milk, cow's milk or coconut milk)

1 small date, pitted and chopped

2 tbsp (14 g) raw cacao powder

2 tbsp (32 g) almond butter

1½ tbsp (15 g) vanilla (or plain) protein powder

Cherry Cacao Smoothie Bowl

This rich and flavorful smoothie bowl is loaded with antioxidants, polyphenols and fiber that your gut loves. With so many topping possibilities, this smoothie is easy to add to your snack or breakfast rotation and you will never grow tired of it! One of the best topping additions for this smoothie bowl is the Cashew Crunch High Fiber Granola (page 125).

Makes 2 smoothie bowls

Combine all ingredients in a blender and blend on high until combined. Add extra milk as needed but keep the consistency thicker than a smoothie. Pour into a bowl and top with your favorite toppings. Eat with a spoon or sip with a straw.

Notes:

Top with: Cashew Crunch High Fiber Granola (page 125), coconut flakes, hemp hearts, cacao nibs, pumpkin seeds or fresh cherries.

To make this even richer, use full-fat coconut cream in place of the almond milk.

To make this into a smoothie use ¼ to ½ cup (60 to 120 ml) more of almond milk.

Gluten Free, Dairy Free, High Fiber, Vegan, Fermented

Classic Hummus Ingredients

1 (15.5-oz [439-g]) can chickpeas, rinsed and drained

½ tsp baking soda

2 lemons, juiced

2 cloves garlic, chopped (or omit if needed)

½ tsp Himalayan salt

½ cup (120 ml) tahini

2–4 tbsp (30–60 ml) ice water, or more as needed

½ tsp ground cumin

1 tbsp (15 ml) extra-virgin olive oil (if omitting garlic, use garlic-infused olive oil)

Beet Hummus

2 steamed and peeled beets

Pumpkin Hummus

¾ cup (180 ml) pumpkin puree

Hummus Trio: Classic, Beet and Pumpkin

This is the creamiest hummus you will ever have! By boiling the chickpeas you not only create the base for the creamy hummus, but you also make the chickpeas easier to digest. You can also use the Sprouted Chickpeas (page 143) to make this hummus even more digestible (skip the boiling if you use sprouted chickpeas).

Hummus is a staple dip in my house because it provides so much fiber, flavor and taste to a meal and each of these hummus variations provides extra flavor and gut loving benefits. Prep this hummus in advance and serve with your favorite grain bowl.

Makes 12 servings

Put the chickpeas and baking soda in a saucepan. Add enough water to cover then place the pan on the stove and bring to a boil. Boil for approximately 20 minutes (or until the chickpeas are soft and the skins are falling off). If you use Sprouted Chickpeas, skip this step.

While the chickpeas are boiling, combine the lemon juice, garlic and salt in a food processor. Let this sit for 10 minutes. After 10 minutes add the tahini and blend until creamy, with no chunks. If the tahini is thick, add 1 tablespoon (15 ml) of hot water at a time until it blends smoothly. If you are adding pumpkin or beets, add these and continue blending until smooth. Be sure to scrape the sides of the processor bowl to allow the entire mixture to blend.

After blending, drizzle in 2 tablespoons (30 ml) of the ice water and make sure the mixture is smooth, pale and creamy. If the tahini is thick, you might need 1 to 2 additional tablespoons (15 to 30 ml) of water.

Strain the boiled chickpeas through a mesh strainer and run cool water over them for 30 seconds. Pat dry and set aside.

Add the cumin and the chickpeas to the food processor. While blending, drizzle in the olive oil. Blend until the mixture is super smooth, about 2 minutes. Scrape the sides of the processor as needed. Add ice water (1 tablespoon [15 ml] at a time) as needed to make super creamy. Add salt and more lemon if desired for extra flavor.

Cover and keep in the fridge for up to 7 days.

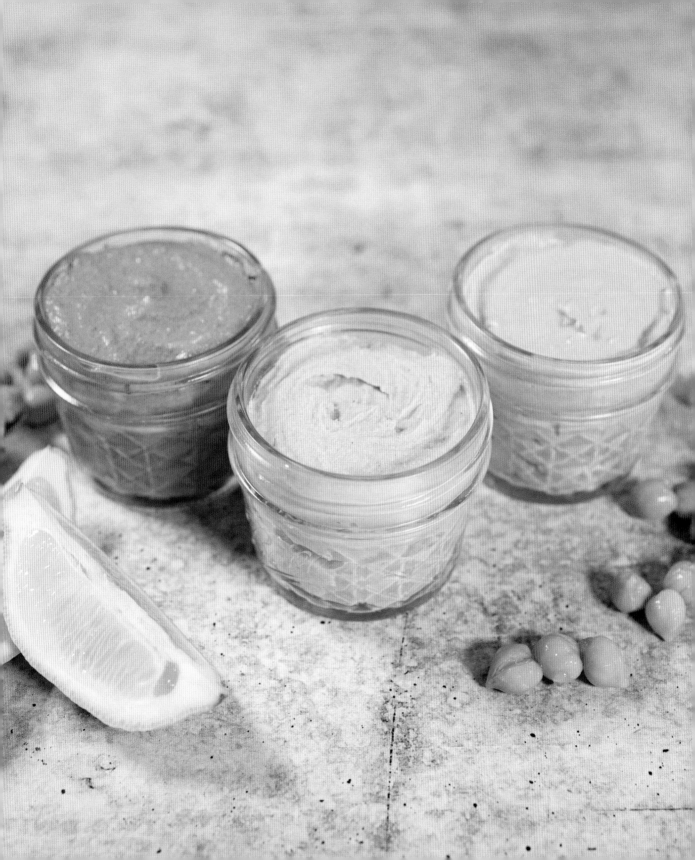

Saucy Additions and
Gut-Loving Toppings

One of the easiest ways to add variety in flavor and nutrition to your meals is through toppings. If you like to meal prep like I do, having extra toppings and sauces on hand can create a completely different meal experience with the same base ingredients. Utilize these toppings and sauces for your favorite biome bowls.

Lemon Tahini Drizzle

2 tbsp (30 ml) warm water

2 tbsp (30 ml) tahini

2 tbsp (30 ml) avocado oil

Juice of 1 lemon (approximately 2–3 tbsp [30–45 ml])

1 clove garlic, minced

½ tsp honey

Lemon Zest Dressing

1 cup (240 ml) olive or avocado oil

Juice and zest of 2 lemons

Salt and pepper, to taste

2 cloves garlic, minced (optional)

Classic Dressing or Marinade

¼ cup (60 ml) apple cider vinegar

¼ cup (60 ml) coconut aminos

2 tbsp (30 ml) avocado oil or olive oil

1 tsp garlic powder

1 tbsp (6 g) pepper

1 tsp onion powder

1 tsp paprika

Salt, to taste

Cilantro–Lime

¼ cup (4 g) fresh cilantro, chopped

2 tbsp (30 ml) avocado or olive oil

Juice and zest of 2 limes

½ tsp chili powder

¼ tsp sea salt

¼ tsp ground black pepper

Saucy Additions

If you are a biome bowl fan, you will also be a fan of sauces that help to switch up the flavor. When your protein, fat, fibrous carbs and fermentation are prepped for your biome bowls, top them off with a delicious sauce. Make one or two at a time so that you have variety in flavor and your gut and your taste buds don't get bored!

Each makes 8 servings

Barbecue Sauce

2 tbsp (32 g) tomato paste

2 tbsp (30 ml) maple syrup

1 tsp garlic powder

1 tsp chili powder

¼ cup (60 ml) coconut aminos

Teriyaki

½ cup (120 ml) coconut aminos

¼ cup (60 ml) maple syrup

2 tbsp (30 ml) apple cider vinegar

2 cloves garlic, minced

2 tsp (10 g) grated fresh ginger

Fresh Herb

¼ cup (15 g) parsley, chopped

¼ cup (4 g) cilantro, chopped

1 tbsp (3 g) chives

1 shallot

2 cloves garlic

½ tsp salt

½ tsp pepper

2 tbsp (30 ml) white wine vinegar

1 tbsp (15 ml) olive oil

For the Lemon Tahini Drizzle, Lemon Zest Dressing, Classic Dressing or Marinade, Cilantro–Lime and Barbecue Sauce, whisk the ingredients together in a bowl or shake together in a jar.

For the Fresh Herb or Teriyaki sauces, blend all the ingredients in a food processor until well combined.

All the sauces will keep in an airtight container in the refrigerator for up to 2 weeks.

Gluten Free, Dairy Free

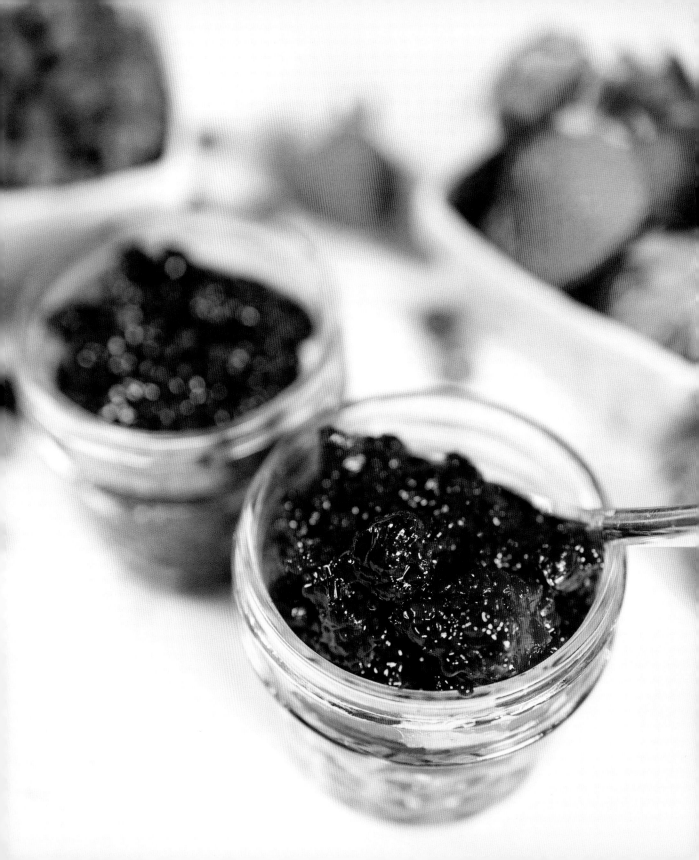

2 cups (375 g) frozen mixed berries

2 tbsp (30 ml) honey, plus more to taste

Juice of 1 lemon

2 tbsp (22 g) chia seeds

Chia Jam

Chia jam makes the perfect addition to your sweet potato pancakes, your sweet potato toast, topping for your overnight oats or even mixed into yogurt. This fiber-, polyphenol- and antioxidant-packed jam is easy to prepare and a fun fiber addition that both you and your gut will love.

Makes 4 servings

Combine all the ingredients in a saucepan over medium heat. Cook, stirring occasionally, until the berries are soft and liquid is evaporated, approximately 20 minutes.

Store in an airtight container in the refrigerator for up to 2 weeks.

Gluten Free, Dairy Free

Pumpkin Seed Pesto

¼ cup (60 ml) olive oil

3 tbsp (21 g) pumpkin seeds

1 clove garlic

2 tbsp (10 g) nutritional yeast

7 basil leaves

Juice of ½ lemon

Salt, to taste

Arugula Pesto

¼ cup (60 ml) olive oil

1 clove garlic

¼ cup (28 g) cashews

Juice of ½ lemon

Salt, to taste

¼ cup (5 g) fresh arugula

Pesto Duo

This pesto duo is a fun, plant-packed and dairy free twist on your traditional pesto. Easy to add to chicken as a dip or on top of your favorite grain bowl, you can whip up these pestos in less than 5 minutes and use for flavor and variety throughout the week.

Both make 4 servings

For either pesto, blend all ingredients in a food processor until smooth. Store in an airtight container in the refrigerator for up to 2 weeks.

Gluten Free, Dairy Free, Vegan

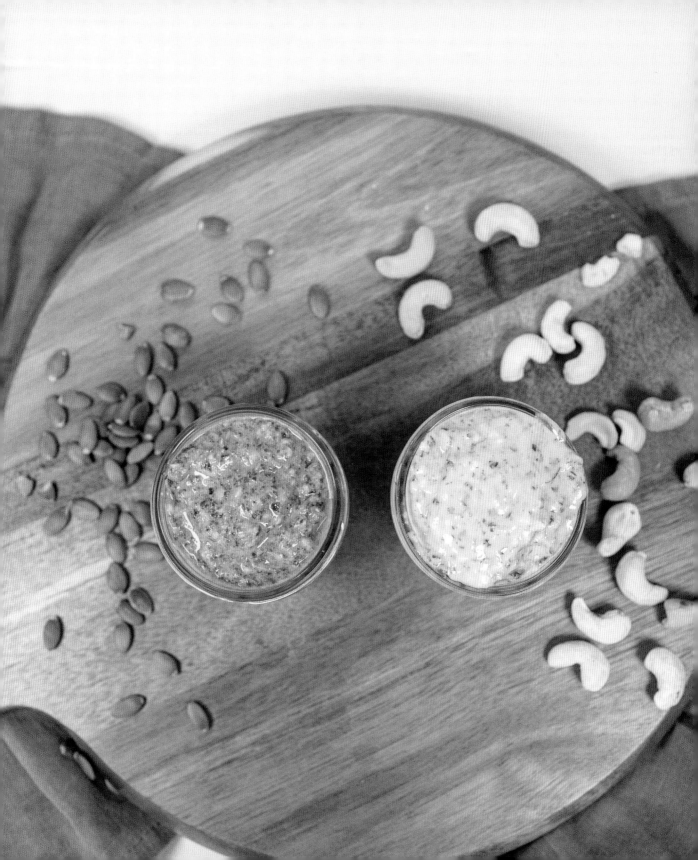

Sprouted
Toppings

Even if you don't have a green thumb, sprouting seeds is easy to do and you don't even need dirt! Sprouting seeds increases the nutrient levels in the seeds, makes the seeds easier to absorb, and creates a fun science experiment right on your kitchen counter. Sprouted seeds are an excellent topping for toast, gut bowls, salads, stir fries and on sandwiches and wraps. Broccoli sprouts are loaded with fiber, sulforaphane for liver detoxification and are rich in vitamins C and A. Chickpea sprouts are high in protein, vitamin C and iron.

½ cup (200 g) chickpeas

1 cup (240 ml) water

Sprouted Chickpeas

Interested in a counter-top science experiment that loves your gut? These chickpea sprouts are easy to make, fun to add as a fiber addition to meals and are easier to digest than traditional chickpeas. The sprouting process increases digestibility by activating enzymes and decreasing phytic acid.

Makes 2 servings

Soak the chickpeas in the water overnight. In the morning, drain the chickpeas and rinse them.

Spread the chickpeas evenly on the bottom of a colander and place the colander over a bowl.

Cover the colander with a dishtowel or paper towels. Rinse and drain the chickpeas two to three times per day. If it is hot, rinse and drain them four to five times per day. Repeat until the chickpeas have sprouted.

If you will be eating the sprouted chickpeas raw, allow the chickpeas to sprout for 5 days.

If you will be using them in a recipe that includes cooking, allow the chickpeas to sprout for 3 days.

When they have sprouted sufficiently, rinse them and drain them. Allow them to air dry before storing in the fridge for up to a week.

Gluten Free, Dairy Free, High Fiber, Vegan

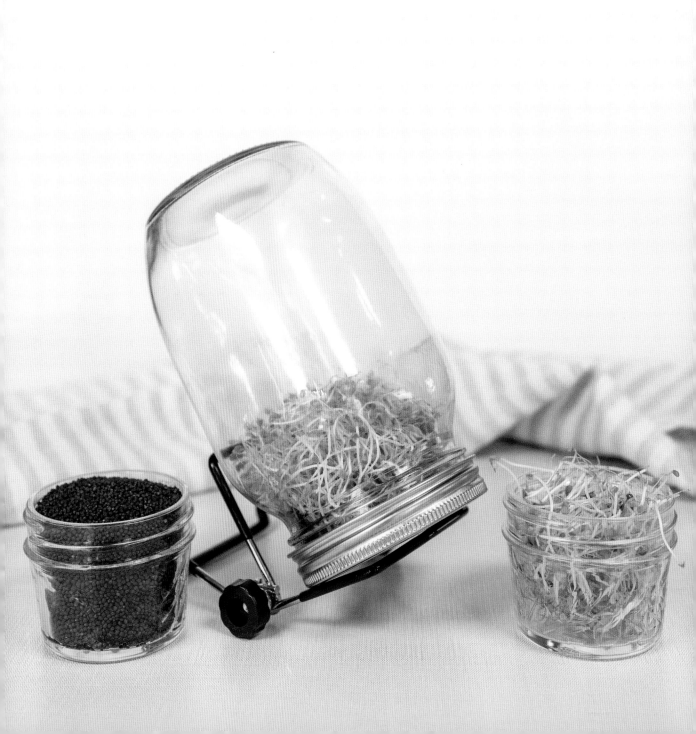

2 tbsp (21 g) broccoli seeds

¼ cup (60 ml) water

Broccoli Sprouts

Broccoli sprouts are one of the easiest and cheapest ways to love your liver and your gut. Broccoli sprouts contain a compound called sulforaphane, which is helpful for liver detoxification and is found in much higher amounts in the sprouts versus the actual vegetable. Grow these sprouts on your counter and always have a fun conversation topic when guests come over to visit. Serve a pinch of these sprouts on your toast, salads, eggs, soups or even blended in smoothies. You'll need a mason jar with a strainer lid; find one online or at a natural food store.

Makes 12 servings

Place the broccoli seeds in a small bowl and add the water. Soak the seeds overnight. In the morning, strain out the water and put the seeds in a mason jar with a strainer lid and turn it upside down so any water remaining can drain.

For 48 hours keep the seeds in a dark, cool place (like your pantry). Be sure to place the mason jar upside down so that the strainer lid will allow any liquid to drain.

Once every 12 hours rinse the seeds and drain the water through the strainer lid.

When the seeds have formed yellow sprouts (on approximately day 4), transfer to a light location (such as your kitchen counter) and continue rinsing every 12 hours. Keep out of direct sunlight. The broccoli sprouts will turn greener during this period.

When the sprouts are nice and green (day 5 or 6) you can give them a final rinse and transfer them to a bowl with a lid. Add a pinch to your salads, tacos, omelets, toast, and more!

Store in the fridge for 5 to 7 days.

Gluten Free, Dairy Free, Vegan, High Fiber

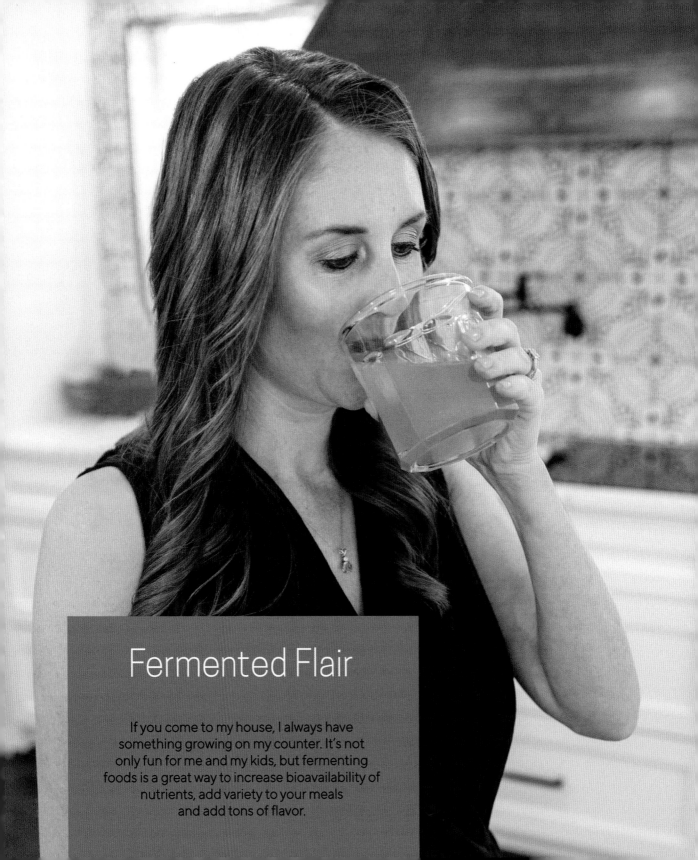

Fermented Flair

If you come to my house, I always have
something growing on my counter. It's not
only fun for me and my kids, but fermenting
foods is a great way to increase bioavailability of
nutrients, add variety to your meals
and add tons of flavor.

1 tbsp (10 g) kefir grains

1 qt (960 ml) milk of choice (cow's milk, coconut milk, goat's milk)

Kefir

Kefir is a probiotic-rich fermented drink that is soon to be a kitchen staple for you! My mother-in-law originally introduced me to kefir when I first met my husband. She continues to provide me kefir grains every time I forget to "feed" mine or stop making it for a while. Kefir is great for smoothies, popsicles and even dips! Because it is fermented, make sure to add it to your diet slowly to build your gut's tolerance. To make this, you will need to find a friend who has kefir grains, or you can purchase them.

Makes 4 servings

Add the kefir grains and the milk to a large mason jar. Cover the jar with a paper towel or coffee filter and secure with a rubber band. Set the jar on the counter for 24 hours. You will know when the kefir is finished when the milk has thickened and smells fermented. Place a non-metal bowl under a fine mesh, non-metal colander. Pour the kefir into the colander to gently force kefir through and leave the grains behind. Rinse the original jar and add the grains back to it.

Store the kefir in the fridge for up to 14 days.

Keep the kefir grains alive by making more kefir or store the grains covered with milk in the fridge for up to 7 days. After 7 days, change the milk and make more kefir, or continue to store.

Gluten Free, Fermented

1 medium head green or purple cabbage

1½ tbsp (22 g) kosher salt

1 tbsp (8 g) caraway seeds

Sauerkraut

Maybe it's my German roots, or my love for gut health, but I absolutely love sauerkraut. On toast, on sandwiches, on salads, on eggs . . . sauerkraut adds a little twist to any meal! It also reminds me of my dad. We used to eat German food every year for his birthday and now instead of eating it once per year, I eat it a couple times a week to continually fuel my gut.

Makes 8 servings (1.5 qt [1.4 L])

Slice the cabbage in half and then into ribbons and transfer to a big bowl. Sprinkle the salt on top. Start massaging the cabbage by squeezing it with your hands. Allow the cabbage to become watery and limp, 5 to 10 minutes. Add the caraway seeds and stir to mix.

Pack the cabbage into a large canning jar. Push the cabbage down with a fist and allow liquid to release. When the cabbage is well packed, put another smaller jar (with stones or marbles inside) on top to weight the cabbage down. Allow the cabbage to be submerged under the liquid. Secure the top of the jar with a cloth and a rubber band.

During the first day, every 4 to 5 hours, press down on the cabbage with the smaller jar and allow the cabbage to become limper. Allow the cabbage to ferment for 3 to 10 days, making sure to keep the jar out of direct sunlight. You will know the sauerkraut is ready when bubbles no longer appear in the liquid. The longer you allow the cabbage to ferment, the tangier the flavor will be.

After it is fermented, store in the fridge for up to a month.

Gluten Free, Dairy Free, Vegan, Fermented

1 cup (240 ml) apple cider vinegar

1 cup (240 ml) water

⅓ cup (66 g) granulated sugar

1 tsp salt

¼ tsp ground mustard

4 medium roasted beets, cooled, peeled, sliced

4 peppercorns (optional)

Pickled Beets

Pickled beets are an easy way to add fermentation and vibrant color to any meal. I especially love pickled beets on tacos, salads and even eggs. Even if you aren't a beet lover, you will love these pickled beets—a pinch on your favorite meal adds just enough sweet and tang.

Makes 16 servings

Bring the vinegar, water, sugar, salt and mustard to a boil in a saucepan. Allow the sugar to dissolve and simmer for 5 minutes. Add the beets and peppercorns to a glass jar. Pour the brine into the jar so that it covers the beets. Set aside and allow the brine to cool slightly. Then, cover with a lid and transfer to the fridge.

These will keep in an airtight container in the refrigerator for up to 6 weeks.

1 qt (960 ml) Kefir (page 147)

1 mini cucumber, thinly sliced (approximately ½ cup [50 g])

2 cloves garlic, minced

2 tbsp (30 ml) lemon juice

2 tbsp (6 g) dill (plus more for garnish, optional)

½ tsp Himalayan sea salt

Parsley, optional, for garnish

Olives, optional, for garnish

Extra virgin olive oil, optional, for garnish

Kefir Tzatziki

If you love Greek food as much as I do, you will love this twist on traditional tzatziki. Greek-inspired biome bowls are a weekly (at least) occurrence for me, and this easy-to-make, fermented topping is a great way to fuel your gut and taste buds. Enjoy this dip as a condiment for a biome bowl or as a dip with pita, crackers or sliced veggies.

Makes 4 servings

Pour the kefir into a cheesecloth (or coffee filter) with a bowl underneath. Let it strain for approximately 6 hours, or until you have approximately 1 cup (240 ml) of very thick kefir (it should be the consistency of Greek yogurt).

Mix the cucumber, garlic, lemon juice, dill and salt into the strained kefir until well combined. Garnish with extra dill, or if desired, parsley, olives or extra virgin olive oil.

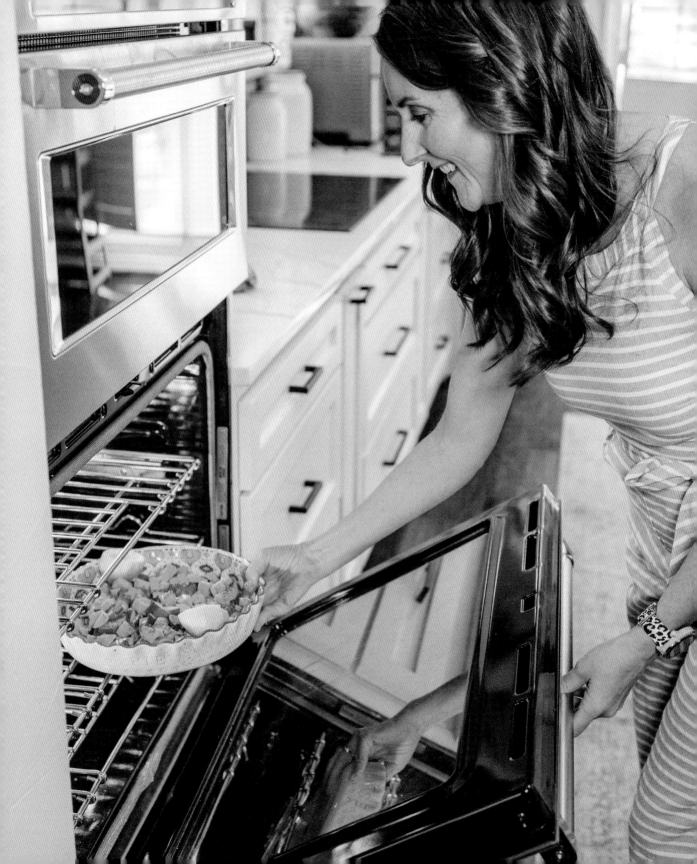

Appendix A: # The Happy Gut Tracker

Habit tracker

DATE _____

MOOD ☹ ☹ 😐 ☺ ☺

today I am *grateful* for:

MEALTIME HABITS	B	L	D
4-7-8 OR BOX BREATHING BEFORE EATING			
PROTEIN SOURCE			
FAT SOURCE			
FIBER SOURCE			
SOMETHING COLORFUL			
CHEWED TO APPLESAUCE CONSISTENCY			
TOOK APPROXIMATELY 20 MINS TO EAT			

Bonus: added a fermented or probiotic-rich food!

MEDS/SUPPLEMENTS TAKEN

circle one

TODAY MY BOWEL MOVEMENTS WERE

1   2   3   4   5   6   7

LIFESTYLE CHECKLIST

- ○ Daily **movement**
- ○ **Motility support** (*gargle 2–3 min, hum or sing*)
- ○ Ended shower in **cold water**
- ○ 15 minutes **stress management**
- ○ **Slept** 7+ hours
- ○ In **bed before 10pm**
- ○ **Neuroplasticity** journal

OTHER NOTES:
symptoms, menstrual cycle, helpful habits, etc.

WATER
drink up!

Check off every time you drink 10oz of water today

○ ○ ○ ○ ○
○ ○ ○ ○ ○

Weekly reflection

what am i *proud of* in the last 7 days:

---

check one

SYMPTOM SCORE (SCORE 1-5)
(1 = no symptoms; 5 = severe)

GAS	1	2	3	4	5
BLOATING	1	2	3	4	5
PAIN	1	2	3	4	5
DIARRHEA	1	2	3	4	5
CONSTIPATION	1	2	3	4	5
NAUSEA	1	2	3	4	5
VOMITING	1	2	3	4	5
Other	1	2	3	4	5

MENSTRUAL STATUS

- ◯ On my period this week
- ◯ About to start my period
- ◯ Just finished my cycle
- ◯ Period is irregular or came at an unexpected time
- ◯ Middle of my cycle
- ◯ Not applicable

AVG HOURS OF SLEEP	AVG BOWEL MOVEMENT TYPE

AVG OZ OF WATER DAILY	AVG ACTIVITY LEVEL

AVG MOOD/ STRESS LEVEL	OVERALL, THIS WEEK WAS

DIVERSITY

fill in!

Every time you eat a plant this week, check off a leaf.
Goal is 30 per week!

Plants include: herbs, spices, nuts, seeds, fruits, vegetables, beans, legumes and whole grains!

MY *smart goal* FOR THIS WEEK IS:

Appendix B: Food Sources of Magnesium

Food sources of magnesium ranked by milligrams of magnesium per standard amount.

Food, Standard Amount	Magnesium (mg)
Pumpkin and squash seed kernels, roasted, 1 oz (28 g)	151
Brazil nuts, 1 oz (28 g)	107
Bran ready-to-eat cereal (100%), ~1 oz (28 g)	103
Halibut, cooked, 3 oz (85 g)	91
Quinoa, dry, ¼ cup (43 g)	89
Spinach, canned, ½ cup (110 g)	81
Almonds, 1 oz (28 g)	78
Spinach, cooked from fresh, ½ cup (95 g)	78
Buckwheat flour, ¼ cup (30 g)	75
Cashews, dry roasted, 1 oz (28 g)	74
Soybeans, mature, cooked, ½ cup (86 g)	74
Pine nuts, dried, 1 oz (28 g)	71
Mixed nuts, oil roasted, with peanuts, 1 oz (28 g)	67
White beans, canned, ½ cup (131 g)	67
Pollock, walleye, cooked, 3 oz (85 g)	62
Black beans, cooked, ½ cup (120 g)	60
Bulgur, dry, ¼ cup (35 g)	57
Oat bran, raw, ¼ cup (23 g)	55
Soybeans, green, cooked, ½ cup (90 g)	54
Tuna, yellowfin, cooked, 3 oz (85 g)	54
Artichokes (hearts), cooked, ½ cup (84 g)	50
Peanuts, dry roasted, 1 oz (28 g)	50
Lima beans, baby, cooked from frozen, ½ cup (90 g)	50
Beet greens, cooked, ½ cup (72 g)	49
Navy beans, cooked, ½ cup (90 g)	48
Tofu, firm, prepared with nigari*, ½ cup (126 g)	47
Okra, cooked from frozen, ½ cup (80 g)	47
Soy beverage, 1 cup (240 ml)	47
Cowpeas, cooked, ½ cup (85 g)	46
Hazelnuts, 1 oz (28 g)	46
Oat bran muffin, 1 oz (28 g)	45
Great Northern beans, cooked, ½ cup (90 g)	44
Oat bran, cooked, ½ cup (120 g)	44
Buckwheat groats, roasted, cooked, ½ cup (84 g)	43
Brown rice, cooked, ½ cup (98 g)	42
Haddock, cooked, 3 oz (85 g)	42

*Calcium sulfate and magnesium chloride.

Source: Nutrient values from Agricultural Research Service (ARS) Nutrient Database for Standard Reference, Release 17.

Appendix C: Neuroplasticity Journal

Today I accept that my digestive symptoms: _____

Morning:

> The things I am grateful for in my life are:

Today I feel inspired to do these things for my digestive health:

1.

2.

3.

I create my day with my thoughts, therefore:

My health is: _____

_____

My gut is: _____

_____

My symptoms are: _____

_____

Evening:

What went well today? _____

_____

What would I like to let go of (regarding my symptoms or something else)? _____

_____

_____

What new habit do I want to adopt? _____

_____

Appendix D:

Gut-Supportive Foods

Foods/beverages containing polyphenols

(This is not an exhaustive list).

Fruits:

- Cranberries
- Cherries
- Blackcurrant
- Apricot
- Peaches
- Pure lemon juice
- Grapes
- Grapefruit
- Pears
- Pomegranate
- Black elderberry
- Apples
- Green olives
- Black olives
- Olive oil
- Strawberries
- Blueberries
- Blackberries
- Raspberries
- Red currants
- Plums
- Nectarine
- Red wine
- White wine
- Avocado

Vegetables:

- Potato
- Carrots
- Capers
- Rapeseed oil
- Onions (red and yellow)
- Kale
- Broccoli
- Endive
- Red lettuce
- Celery
- Artichoke (globe artichoke heads)
- Spinach
- Shallot
- Asparagus

Beans/legumes:

- White beans
- Soybeans including tempeh and tofu and soy milk (try for organic, non-GMO)
- Cocoa including dark chocolate (the darker the better, opt for 70% or higher)
- Black beans

Whole grains:

- Whole wheat flour
- Whole grain rye flour
- Whole grain oat flour
- Oats

Nuts/seeds:

- Pecans
- Almonds
- Hazelnuts
- Flaxseeds
- Walnuts
- Sesame seeds

Beverages:

- Green tea
- Black tea
- Chicory (green and red chicory) → great replacement for coffee
- Organic soy milk (non-GMO)
- Organic coffee

Herbs/spices:

- Cloves
- Anise
- Peppermint
- Oregano
- Cinnamon
- Ginger
- Celery seed
- Sage
- Thyme
- Rosemary
- Spearmint
- Basil
- Curry powder
- Lemon verbena
- Cumin
- Caraway
- Parsley

Foods high in vitamin A (helpful for low immunoglobulin A levels and gut immune system):

- Liver (beef and lamb)
- Carrots
- Tuna
- Butternut squash
- Sweet potato
- Pumpkin
- Acai berries
- Bluefin tuna
- Spinach
- Cantaloupe
- Lettuce
- Red bell peppers
- Pink grapefruit
- Broccoli

Foods high in vitamin D (helpful for gut immune system and hormones; you may need to take a supplement if your levels are very low or you live in a cloudy area):

- Salmon
- Herring and sardines
- Cod liver oil
- Canned tuna
- Egg yolks
- Mushrooms

Foods fortified with vitamin D (it is best to get your vitamin D from non-fortified sources):

- Cow's milk
- Orange juice
- Soy milk
- Cereal and oatmeal

Foods high in vitamin C (helpful for immune support):

- Guavas
- Kiwi
- Bell peppers
- Strawberries
- Oranges
- Papaya
- Broccoli
- Tomato
- Snow peas
- Kale

Foods high in omega-3s (helpful for inflammation):

- Salmon
- Mackerel
- Tuna
- Herring
- Sardines
- Omega-3 eggs

Vegetarian sources:

- Chia: high in fiber and omegas, soak for better digestibility
- Flax (get ground flaxseeds for better digestibility)
- Flaxseed oil is also a great source
- Hemp (high in protein)
- Walnuts (soak for easier digestibility)
- Algae oil (mostly found in supplement form)
- Perilla oil (can be used as a flavor enhancer in dressing)

Foods high in zinc (helpful for digestive enzyme production and stomach acid production; also helpful for tight junction support):

- Oysters
- Beef shanks
- Crab, Alaska king
- Pork shoulder and pork tenderloin
- Lobster
- Roasted chicken leg and/or breast with skin removed

- Baked beans
- Cashews, dry roasted
- Chickpeas
- Cheese (Swiss, Cheddar, or mozzarella)
- Almonds, dry roasted
- Milk, whole
- Kidney beans
- Pumpkin seeds
- Foods containing resistant starch
- Cooked and cooled oats
- Cooked and cooled rice
- Cooked and cooled sorghum and barley
- Beans and legumes
- Raw potato starch
- Cooked and cooled potatoes
- Green bananas
- HI-MAIZE® resistant starch

Appendix E: Soaking and Sprouting Guide

Benefits of Soaking and Sprouting:

- Increases digestibility
- Increases nutrient bioavailability
- Reduces phytic acid content
- Increases fiber content

Soaking 101

Step 1: Fill

Fill one-third of a container with your chosen nut, seed, bean or legume.

Step 2: Add water

Fully submerge the substance with warm water and a pinch of sea salt.

Step 3: Soak

Cover the container and let the substance soak for the required time. See page 158 for soaking times.

Step 4: Drain and rinse

Drain and rinse; cook, consume or dehydrate within 24 hours.

Step 5: Sprout (optional)

After draining and rinsing, leave the container open to allow air circulation; rinse twice a day until sprouts appear. After rinsing, refrigerate in an airtight container.

Soaking and Sprouting Times:

Nuts

- **Almonds:** 2–12 hours for soaking, sprout for 2–3 days if raw
- **Walnuts:** 4 hours soaking, do not sprout
- **Brazil nuts:** 3 hours soaking, do not sprout
- **Cashews:** 2–3 hours soaking, do not sprout
- **Hazelnuts:** 8 hours soaking, do not sprout
- **Macadamias:** 2 hours soaking, do not sprout
- **Pecans:** 6 hours soaking, do not sprout
- **Pistachios:** 8 hours soaking, do not sprout

Beans and legumes

- **Chickpeas:** 8–12 hours soaking, 2–3 days for sprouting
- **Lentils:** 8 hours soaking, 2–3 days for sprouting
- **Adzuki beans:** 8 hours soaking, 2–3 days for sprouting
- **Black beans:** 8–12 hours soaking, 3 days for sprouting
- **White beans:** 8 hours soaking, 2–3 days for sprouting
- **Mung beans:** 24 hours soaking, 2–5 days for sprouting
- **Kidney beans:** 8–12 hours soaking, 5–7 days for sprouting
- **Navy beans:** 9–12 hours soaking, 2–3 days for sprouting
- **Peas:** 9–12 hours soaking, 2–3 days for sprouting

Grains

- **Buckwheat:** 30 minutes–6 hours soaking (time varies), 2–3 days for sprouting
- **Amaranth:** 8 hours soaking, 1–3 days for sprouting
- **Kamut:** 7 hours soaking, 2–3 days for sprouting
- **Millet:** 8 hours soaking, 2–3 days for sprouting
- **Oat groats:** 6 hours soaking, 2–3 days for sprouting
- **Quinoa:** 4 hours soaking, 1–3 days for sprouting
- **Wheat berries:** 7 hours soaking, 3–4 days for sprouting
- **Wild rice:** 9 hours soaking, 3–5 days for sprouting
- **Black rice:** 9 hours soaking, 3–5 days for sprouting

Seeds

- **Radish seeds:** 8–12 hours soaking, 3–4 days for sprouting
- **Alfalfa seeds:** 12 hours soaking, 3–5 days for sprouting
- **Pumpkin seeds:** 8 hours soaking, 1–2 days for sprouting
- **Sesame seeds:** 8 hours soaking, 1–2 days for sprouting
- **Sunflower seeds:** 8 hours soaking, 2–3 days for sprouting
- Flax, chia and hemp seeds are difficult to sprout so most people avoid trying this. However, you can sprout these small seeds by following the directions on page 159
- Macadamia nuts and pine nuts also normally don't need to be sprouted unless the recipe tells you to do so
- It's not recommended to sprout red kidney beans

To sprout chia, hemp and flaxseeds:

Sprouting small seeds is a different process than that of most larger seeds from nuts, grains, beans and legumes. Smaller seeds form a mucilaginous coat that gives them a gel-like consistency when soaked in water. They can't be sprouted using the usual method and do better when sprouted in a shallow dish, such as terracotta, clay or ceramic dishes or trays.

1. Fill a shallow dish with a slight amount of water. Add about a teaspoon or so of seeds. Let the seeds soak for several minutes, then drain them.

2. Sprinkle your seeds back onto the dish. They should be evenly spread and only in a single layer. There should be space between seeds to allow them to spread while growing. Cover with clear glass or a plastic bowl. Place in a sunny spot.

3. Spray the dish twice a day with a small amount of water. Try to keep the surface of the dish wet at all times if possible. The seeds absorb water and plump up, so keep them moist. The sprouts should take 3 to 7 days to appear. They will be about ½ to ¾ inches (1.3 to 2 cm) high when they're ready.

Appendix F: Protein, Fat, Fibrous Carbs and Color

Protein:

- 4 oz (113 g) chicken
- 2–3 chicken legs
- 1 chicken breast
- 1 chicken thigh
- 1–2 chicken sausages
- 4 oz (113 g) fish
- ½ cup (113 g) cottage cheese
- 5 large shrimp
- 9 medium scallops
- 4 large scallops
- 1 jerky stick
- 2 eggs
- 4 oz (113 g) steak
- 4 oz (113 g) crab
- 4 oz (113 g) chorizo
- ½ cup (120 ml) Greek yogurt
- 1–2 slices nitrate-free deli meat
- 2 egg whites

Plant-based protein:

- 1 scoop (1½ tbsp [15 g]) protein powder
- 4 oz (113 g) tofu
- 4 oz (113 g) tempeh
- ½ cup (100 g) cooked lentils, chickpeas, beans or legumes
- ½ cup (80 g) cooked green peas
- ½ cup (55 g) cooked edamame

Fat:

- 1 oz (28 g) chia seeds
- 2 tbsp (17 g) sunflower seeds
- 1 tbsp (16 g) nut butter
- ¼ cup (40 g) nuts
- 6 macadamia nuts
- 12 hazelnuts
- 25 pistachios

Oils:

- 1 tsp (5 g) ghee/butter
- 1 tbsp (15 ml) olive oil/coconut oil/avocado oil

Other:

- ¼ avocado
- ¼ cup (60 ml) full-fat coconut milk
- 2 tbsp (30 ml) mayo
- 2 tbsp (30 ml) hummus
- 2 tbsp (30 ml) guacamole
- 10 olives
- 1 piece cheese (3 dice-sized pieces)
- 1 tbsp (15 ml) coconut cream
- 1 tbsp (16 g) dark chocolate

Fiber/Carbs:

Colorful carbs:

- ½ cup fruit
- ⅓ cup (70 g) cooked squash
- ½ sweet potato
- ⅓ cup (53 g) cooked peas
- 1 tbsp (9 g) raisins
- ½ cup (70 g) cooked or raw carrots
- ½ potato
- 1 cup (150 g) cooked or raw bell peppers

Fibrous grains:

- ½ cup (93 g) cooked quinoa
- ½ cup (100 g) cooked beans
- ½ cup (80 g) cooked rice
- ½ cup (87 g) cooked millet
- 8 rice crackers
- ⅓ cup (32 g) almond flour
- 1 rice cake
- ⅓ cup (50 g) cooked corn
- ½ cup (84 g) cooked buckwheat
- ¼ cup (28 g) coconut flour

Color:

- Any fruit or vegetable
- **Note:** sometimes the fiber/carb will overlap with the color (e.g., if you are eating sweet potatoes as your carb). In that case, add some greens as your color!

Bristol Stool Scale

Use this chart to rate your bowel movements each day. The ratings tell you a lot about what's going on!

Type 1		Separate hard lumps that are hard to pass
Type 2		Sausage shaped, but lumpy
Type 3		Like a sausage but with cracks on the surface
Type 4		Smooth, soft log like a snake or sausage
Type 5		Soft blobs with clear-cut edges
Type 6		Fluffy pieces with ragged edges, a very mushy stool
Type 7		Watery, no solid pieces

Acknowledgments

Writing a book has been a dream of mine for more than a decade. In 2012, I promised my dad before he lost his battle with colon cancer that I would write a book to help other people—it was one of the last conversations that we had. At that time, I had no idea where my career path would take me as I was still a very new registered dietitian; but here we are 10 years later, and I am so grateful to have had this opportunity. Although I would give anything to have him back here to physically read this book, I am thankful for his influence on my life and his encouragement to always pursue my dreams. He was one of my biggest cheerleaders. In his honor I plan to donate some of the proceeds of this book to colon cancer research.

I also want to thank the following people for always pushing me to dream bigger . . .

To my husband, for being the ultimate hype man and for always pushing me to take big risks. I wouldn't be here today without you. Your support, encouragement and loyalty mean the world to me.

My mom, your strength and courage inspire me. Thank you for teaching me to love the kitchen and instilling in me a love for nourishing others with food.

Leah and Max, thank you for being my test subjects, even when you didn't want to be!

Pat and Barb, my wonderful in-laws, thank you for always loaning me kefir grains when I forget to feed mine! Thank you also for your willingness to help at the drop of a hat.

Ellie, my ride or die—thank you for always being willing to brainstorm with me at the drop of a hat. We talked about this book more than a decade ago and I cannot believe it's actually happening.

To the entire Page Street Publishing team, thank you for trusting me with this opportunity. I am forever grateful.

Finally, to my precious kids. Charlotte, you are the best "cookbook helper" and recipe taster. I always appreciate your honest, toddler feedback. Weldon, you experienced writing this book both inside and outside of the womb. It will always be one of our greatest adventures. May you both always dream bigger, as you have both taught me to do. I will always be there to cheer you on.

About the Author

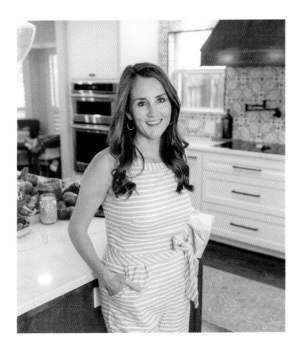

Dr. Heather Finley is the founder and registered dietitian behind the gutTogether method and the gutPractitioner program. Dr. Heather struggled with her own digestive issues for nearly 20 years and understands firsthand the impact that nutrition, lifestyle and mindset have on digestive health. Dr. Heather strives to make gut health approachable and achievable so that individuals can reduce stress and fear around food, find joy in the kitchen again and live life vibrantly again (sans the digestive symptoms). Dr. Heather lives in the Dallas-Fort Worth area with her husband Dave and two children, Charlotte and Weldon.

Dr. Heather is a contributing writer to several health and wellness organizations, as well as a speaker and mentor to other health professionals. You can find her educating audiences on gut health and nutrition both online and at in-person seminars. She received a bachelor of science in nutrition from Texas Christian University, a master's in kinesiology from Texas Christian University and a doctorate in clinical nutrition from Maryland University of Integrative Health.

Index